Coconut Oil

Coconut oil cures including virgin coconut oil for weight loss, coconut oil for hair and other coconut oil benefits

Ellen Vincent

First Printing, 2012

ISBN - 13: 978-1481261838

ISBN - 10: 1481261835

Printed in the United States of America

Dedication

For my family in Ghana

Coconut Oil

Table of Contents

Introduction 9
The importance of using virgin coconut oil 13
Making your own cold pressed virgin coconut oil 17
Hair care with coconut oil 23
Treating head lice 31
Caring for your skin with coconut oil 35
Mouth care with coconut oil 41
Acne control using coconut oil 43
Coconut oil for weight loss 47
Coconut oil cures for digestion problems 53
Immunity and fighting against infections 57
Fight off Candida with coconut oil 61
Coconut oil and type 2 diabetes 65
Coconut oil to prevent heart disease 69
Alzheimer's and dementia treatment 73
Anti cancer properties of coconut oil 83
Conclusion 85
About the Author 89

Introduction

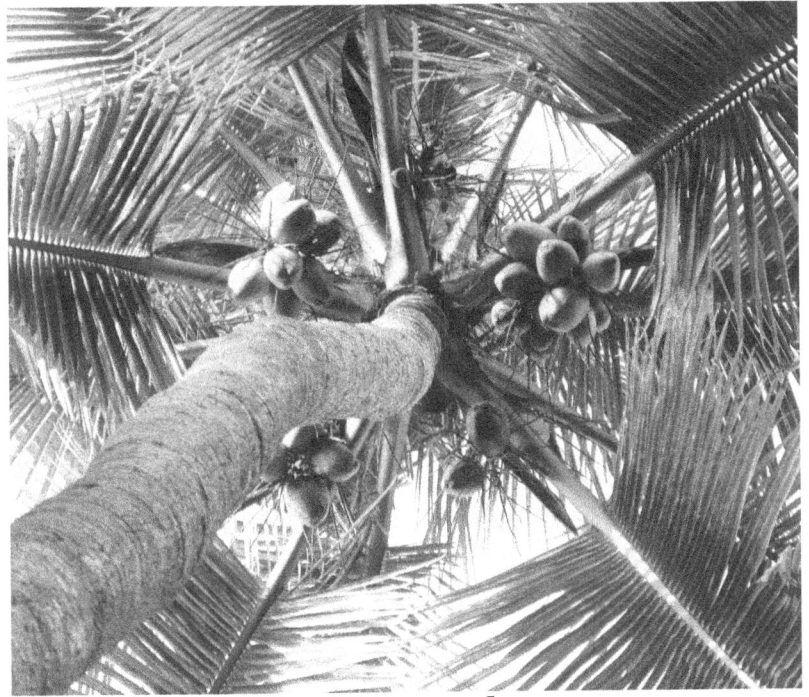

Coconuts on a palm tree

To most of us coconuts and coconut trees are exotic things that we only seem to come into contact with when we are on holiday. However, coconut foods and products are exported across the world these days and you will find them at your local market, supermarket and local health food shops. I even bought a fresh coconut, with the green husk still on, from our local market just the other day.

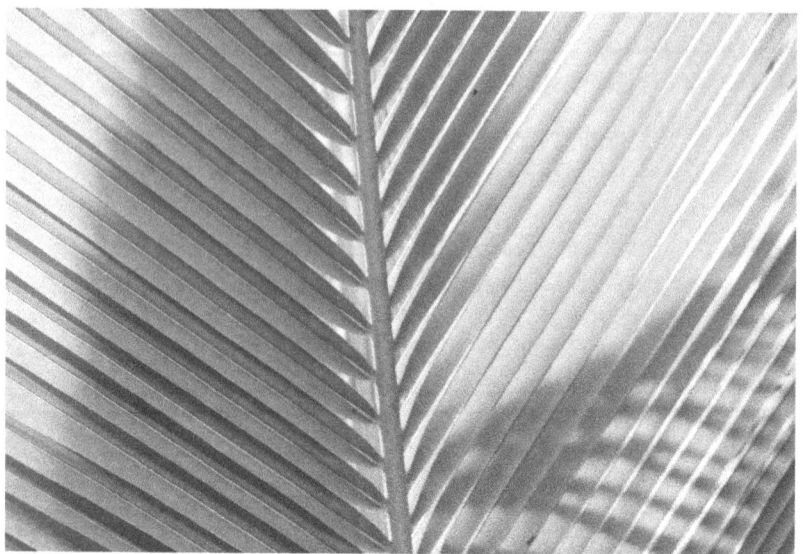
Palm leaves used for construction

People in African countries certainly know the value of the coconut tree and when I visit Ghana I see that coconut leaves are used for roof coverings, the husks are used to make mats and the shells are used for making bowls. Fresh coconut water is used as a refreshing drink in Ghana and is found on most street corners. The seller just chops off the end with his cutlass and away you go. I noticed last week that our health food shop had cartons of coconut water and were advertising the refreshing and health giving values of the drink. In addition to this, creamed coconut made from the fleshy inside of the coconut, has been used for centuries in traditional Asian and Indian cuisine.

There has been a great interest in the health benefits of coconut oil and this has lead to its addition to many creams and other beauty products. There are also many recipes that it has been added to, in order to supply its health giving properties to the body. The oil is therefore often used as a substitute for other oils that have proved to be less healthy for the body.

Despite all of the excited activity surrounding coconut oil there is still a lot of confusion as to whether health claims for coconut oil have been blown out of proportion. Added to this is the fact that based on all of the things we are usually told about oils, coconut oil shouldn't be in the list of healthy ones. This book explores the evidence related to the health claims about coconut oil and tries to explain why, despite all of the usual advice about oils, fats and diet, coconut should still be considered as a valuable tool in keeping our bodies healthy. In doing this we have to separate the myth from reality and try to think about oils and fats in a totally new way.

The importance of using virgin coconut oil

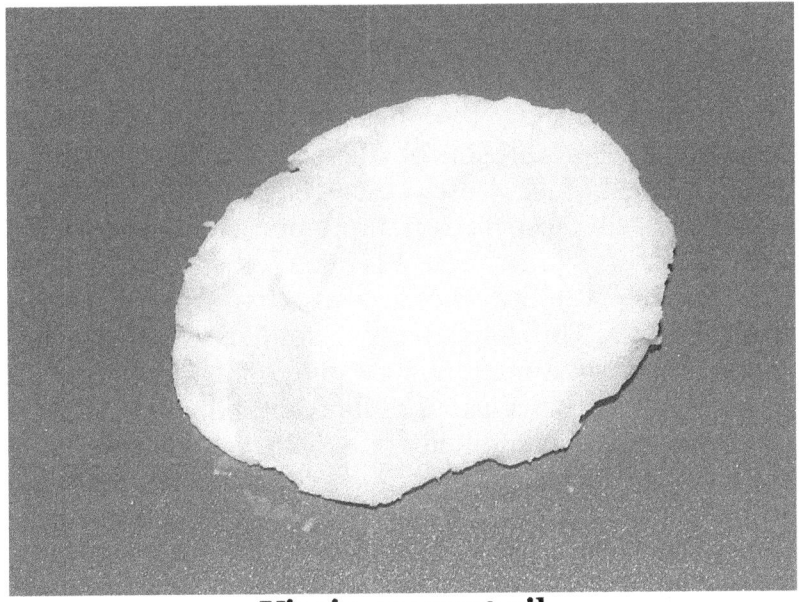

Virgin coconut oil

Virgin coconut oil is the good stuff. It contains all of the important nutrients that are good for the health of your body. It is best obtained from fresh coconut flesh rather than the dried kind. To get the oil out of the coconut it is minced and then mixed with water. This allows the water to mix with the oil and form an emulsion. Ordinary cow's milk is an emulsion and is a white color because of the fat that is suspended in it. The coconut emulsion would look the same white color as milk and as a result this stage is often called coconut milk. In the coconut oil industry, to get the coconut oil out of this emulsion they have to use a centrifuge after first filtering to remove any solid matter. As the centrifuge spins the mixture separates into two layers with oil floating on the water molecules. It is then relatively easy to remove the top layer of coconut oil by skimming it.

The liquid extracted, by this method, is the virgin coconut oil and it is this that contains all of the good nutrients that your body requires. The main important ingredients in this oil are a group of substances called Medium Chain Triglycerides or MCT for short. This MCT is broken down in the body during the digestion process. Digestion results in the production of Medium Chain Fatty Acids being formed. These are often referred to as MCFA. MCFA is easily absorbed by the blood capillaries in the small intestine and from here is taken directly to the liver. Once in the liver the MCFA is used to produce energy straight away. This happens in a similar way to glucose which is the usual main energy source for the body. In a way, the MCFA behaves more like a carbohydrate than a fat in the way that the body uses it in metabolism. Long chain fatty acids from other fats and oils have to be acted on by bile salts and lipase enzymes in the small intestine before they can be absorbed into the lymphatic system. The medium chain fatty acids from coconut oil need far less processing before they can be used in the body.

Virgin Coconut oil had been used for centuries by indigenous peoples where the plants actually grow. It was originally looked on as being a viable substitute for all of the vegetable oils and animal fats that we use for cooking in the Western countries. Unfortunately, there was a need for obtaining more of the coconut oil and as a result companies started using dried coconut as well. The method of extracting the oil from dried coconut was a lot more difficult and resulted in a product that was of a poorer quality. To deal with this situation they put the product through another process. This process is called hydrogenation and resulted in making the fats in the oil more saturated. It also resulted in the production of trans fatty acids as well. This has the effect of changing the coconut oil into something that has more of the properties of animal fats. These are of course the fats that health professionals have been so concerned about in the Western diet. Trans fatty acids also have a bad name. Both of these fats have been identified as causing the clogging of arteries during atherosclerosis. This in turn can cause coronary heart disease. The net result is that a useful healthy natural product was converted into a similar product that was totally unhealthy. For this reason you should make sure that the Coconut oil that you buy is of the virgin type rather than the hydrogenated version. There is also an idea that other vegetable oil producers feared that they would lose out to the new better coconut product and as a result waged a war against it by over emphasizing the bad news about the hydrogenated version. The benefits of raw coconut oil were then neatly swept under the carpet. Despite losing out to the more popular vegetable oils it is encouraging to find that more and more people are turning to coconut oil once again.

Making your own cold pressed virgin coconut oil

Although you can buy virgin coconut oil from health shops and the internet you may wish to try and make your own. This is a relatively simple process but don't expect to get huge amount of oil from your coconuts. It is also a satisfying experience to go through the processes and end up with your own oil.

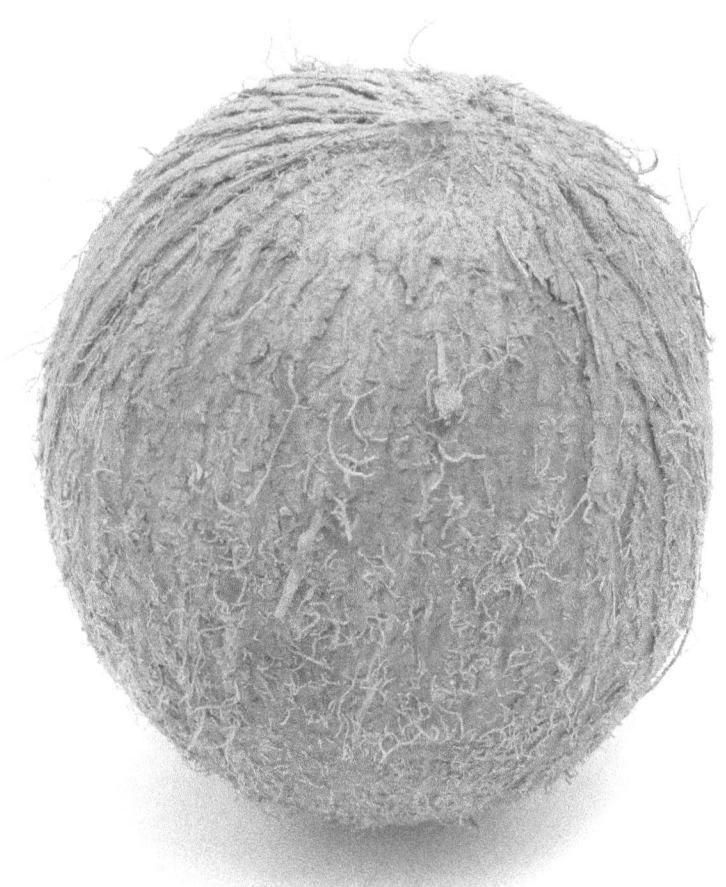

A mature coconut

The first thing to do is to get some mature coconuts. These are the ones that are brown on the outside and contain a thick layer of hard white flesh on the inside. It is the flesh that you need and younger less mature coconuts won't have as much flesh inside them. Once you have the coconuts drain off the coconut water. You can push a hole through the softer eye looking patches on the one end of the coconut.

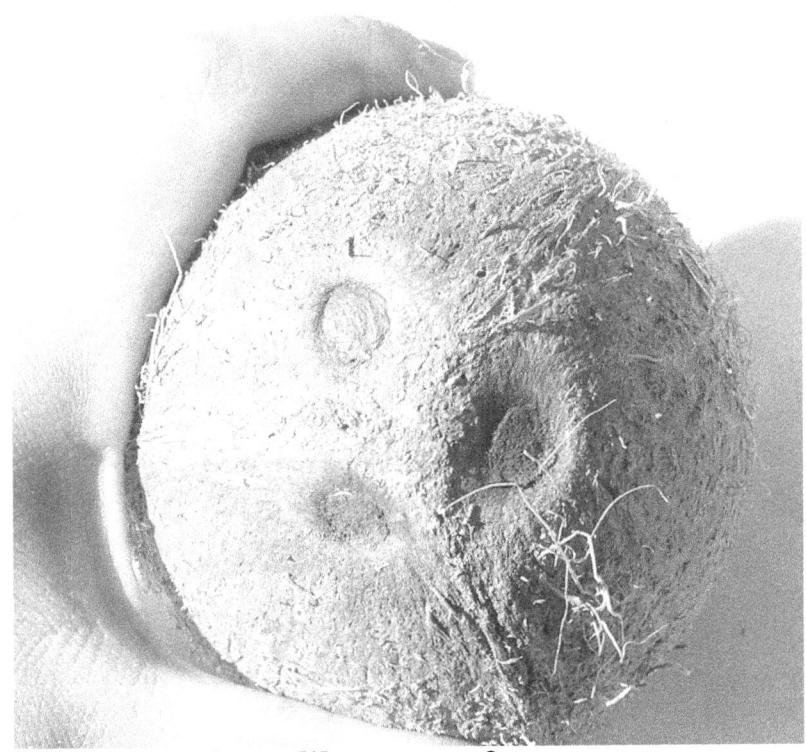

Soft eye like areas of a coconut

Make 2 holes and drain of the water inside the coconut. You can keep this as a refreshing drink to be used on its own or to dilute fruit juices. Wrap the drained coconut in a towel or clean piece of cloth and bash with a hammer or something heavy to smash it open. In mature coconuts the flesh is hard and stuck to the inside of the shell of the nut. Use a knife to push under the coconut flesh and prize it away from the shell. You may find this easier to do if you score the flesh with a sharp knife down to the shell first and then try to remove smaller chunks of the flesh with the knife.

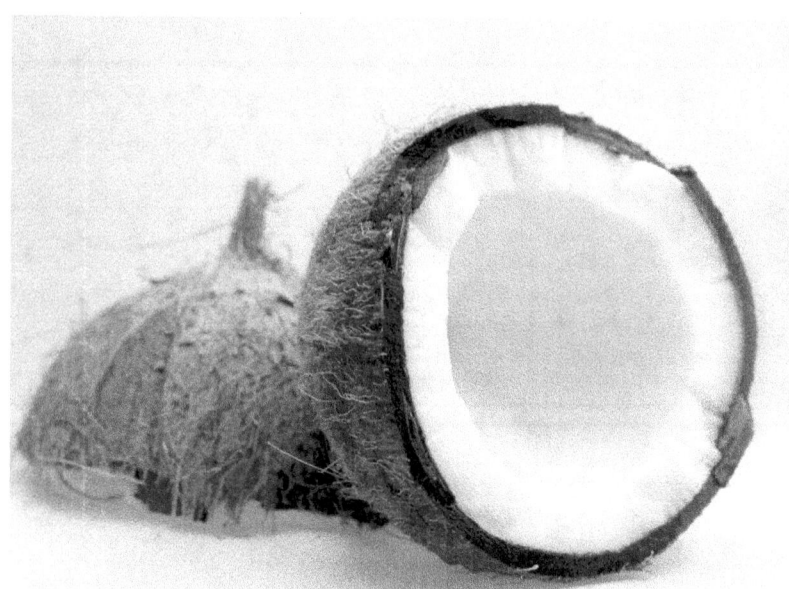

Remove the white flesh from the inside of the coconut

Once you have the flesh separated from the hard shell you need to shred it into smaller bits. To do this you can use a hand grater, if you don't mind some hard work. Alternatively you can put the large chunks of flesh into a blender or food processor. Use the pulse feature of the blender to get it started. If the blender blades won't work on the flesh you should add a little water until the blades pull in the flesh and start to rip it up. Use the blend or chop feature of those blenders with program buttons.

Once the coconut is nice and shredded pour it into a large bowl. Add some water, if it appears to be too dry. You need water for the oil to pass into and form the coconut milk. In order to get the oil to come out of the shredded coconut put your hands into the bowl and grab handfuls of the coconut and squeeze it. This will then help to press the oil out of the coconut flesh. Continue to do this until the water around the coconut has gone very milky.

Next you need to separate the milk from the sold coconut pieces and you should use a fine sieve or a piece of fine muslin cloth. With your hand squeeze the milk out of the coconut pieces and allow it to collect into a separate bowl. You can put the shredded coconut back into water again and try to extract some more of the oil by repeating the process in the last paragraph. Put the coconut milk that you have made into the refrigerator and leave it over night. The pure coconut oil will collect on the surface of the water and you can then skim it off the water using a spoon the next morning. While the coconut oil is cold and solid you can put it into a fine sieve so that the excess water drains off. You should ideally leave it to do this in the refrigerator so that the oil remains solid. Once you have the oil on its own transfer it to a glass jar with a lid and store it away from sunlight in a nice cool place. Some people use jars made out of dark glass to help prevent the sun from affecting it. The oil should keep as long as the shop bought stuff but I dare say that you will have used the coconut oil that you have made within a few days! You can use it for cooking or for any of the other purposes detailed in this book.

Hair care with coconut oil

Coconut oil acts as a super conditioner for hair. Coconut oil is the one oil that our hair can absorb better than any other. The great benefit of this oil is that it is a purely natural product. A lot of women have noticed that conditioners with added artificial ingredients can have a damaging effect on the hair and the scalp when used over long periods of time. This is particularly so as far as black African hair is concerned. Here the hair and scalp can react badly to such substances as paraben preservatives, alcohol and many petroleum derived substances. Just take a look at the conditioner that you usually use, if it contains any of these substances then you may be doing more harm than good by using it.

Another good reason for using coconut oil is that it is relatively cheap, considering the great results that it produces. The coconut oil helps your hair in many ways from: keeping it totally moisturized; allowing the hair to grow fully; producing hair that is strong and won't break easily through to preventing dandruff flakes from developing. One of the ways that it makes your hair stronger and fuller is by maintaining the quality of the protein keratin that makes up your hair.

A large number of commercial cosmetic companies have started to recognize the importance of coconut oil when it comes to conditioning hair but their response has been to add relatively small amounts of it to their products and then still adding the artificial petroleum based substances as well. This means that the benefits of the coconut oil are often outweighed by these other chemicals. This does however allow them to claim that their product is superior because it does in fact contain some coconut oil.

Coconut oil has often been given as a remedy for hair loss. This is especially true where hair has stopped growing at the hair line. This loss can often be due to the use of harsh chemicals to treat hair. Examples of these are hair relaxers and hair perm solutions. My sister used to use a lot of these, but since using coconut oil as a conditioner her hair has started to regrow, but not only that, it has grown a lot stronger as well.

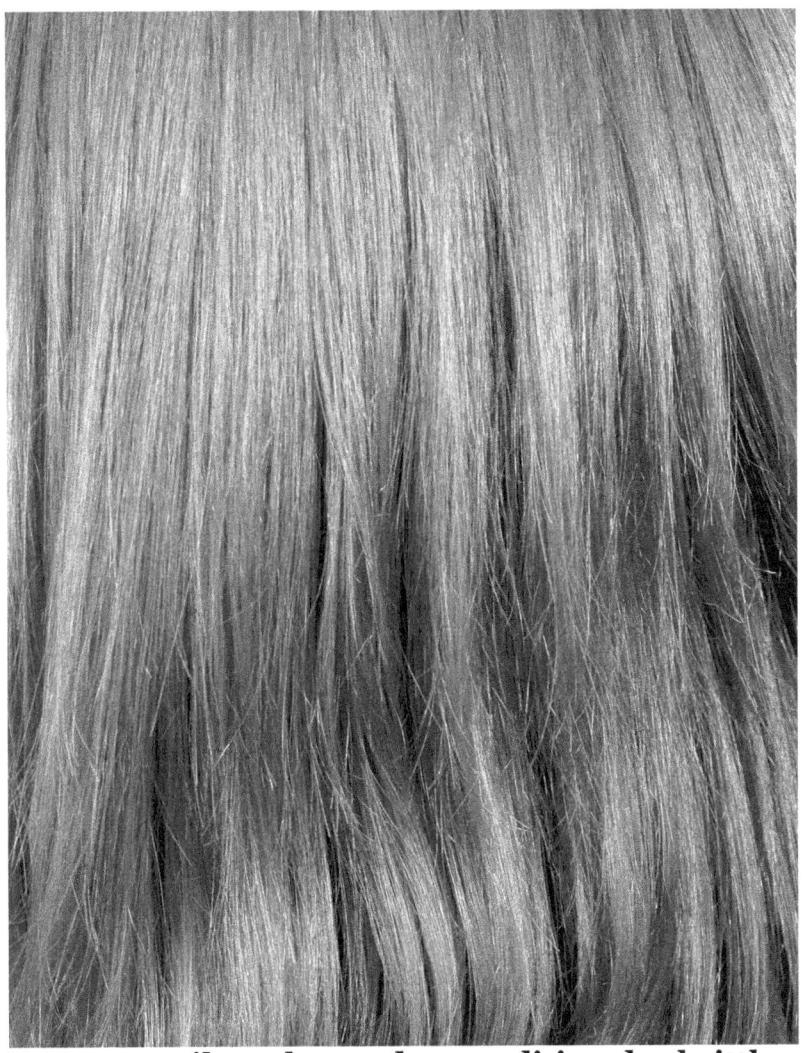

Coconut oil can be used to condition dry brittle hair

Coconut oil is a great choice when it comes to dealing with brittle dry hair. Most commercial hair moisturizers only put a temporary shine on your dry hair. They won't actually deal with the real problem of the dry hair. The reason for this is that they can't actually get into the hair shaft. Moisturizers based on lanolin and mineral oils only coat the hair and give the impression that it has actually been moisturized. Water based products do a little better but they tend to let you down if the hair is relaxed or heat styled later. The only really effective hair moisturizer is virgin coconut oil. This is because it can penetrate right into the shaft and core of every strand of your hair.

You can use virgin coconut oil as a daily moisturizer for your hair. To do this, take a little of the oil and rub it into the palm of your hand. It will start to melt as soon as it touches the skin. Start to rub the oil throughout your hair. Concentrate on the strands of hair rather than the scalp. Always start with a small amount of oil because if you use too much the hair will become greasy and heavy. With this in mind, you can use this method to moisturize you hair as often as needed.

You can use virgin coconut oil as a prewash in order to really get the moisture into your hair. The first thing to do is to get a big handful of coconut oil out of your jar. With long hair you should bend down forwards and flip your hair forward. Start to spread the oil slowly through your hair. The oil will start to melt as soon as it touches your skin and spread into your hair so there is no need to heat the oil before you use it. Make sure that the oil is massaged into all of the hair and concentrate on those parts that you know are problem dry areas. Once you have done this, and all of your hair is soaked in coconut oil, you should tie it up into a ponytail or a bun. Clip or tie your hair up in this position.

Use a shower cap to cover your hair and leave the oil to soak in for about thirty minutes. You can do the job more quickly by applying heat to the shower cap using a hair dryer. The heat helps the coconut oil get into the hair more quickly. If you use heat you will need to heat it for at least fifteen minutes. After the time is up you should wash your hair and condition it as you usually would.

If the hair is still too oily you may need to wash it twice. Concentrate on washing the roots and only do just enough to the ends of the hair where you want the oil to do its magic work. You can then go on to style your hair and be generally stunned as to how smooth and soft your hair is, after applying the coconut oil. If your hair is in bad shape you will need to apply the oil each time you wash it. As the condition of the hair improves you can back off to a regular treatment of once a week. If you maintain the treatment you will find that your hair will grow both longer and stronger.

Hair is rather like a tube and as such is hollow inside. This is often called the hair shaft. Coconut oil is a natural product and has water loving chemical groups as part of its makeup. This means that it is ideally made to get into the hair shaft and fill it up. This then gives the hair more body and makes it look full and thick.

During normal hair treatments such as washing and styling, the hair fibers are subjected to alternate swelling and shrinking. This is due to alternate water absorption, retention and loss. This is a type of hair fatigue. Coconut helps to prevent this because once it has penetrated the core of the hair it prevents it swelling up. This is the reason why coconut oil helps to protect your hair even during heat treatments.

Hair is made up from protein and these proteins can be lost from the hair. This causes damage and weakness to the hair. Regular moisturizing with coconut oil helps to stop the protein being lost from your hair. Coconut oil will seal the hair from the outside and this means that moisture is kept in the hair. This means that it will have a shiny and silky feel to it. The coconut oil in the shaft of the hair can move down into the hair follicle where it supplies moisture. This helps to protect it from heat damage due to styling and chemical damage from other hair treatments.

Coconut oil contains some specific substances which have been identified as being very good for the health and growth of hair. These are all natural substances and are found in useful amounts in coconut oil.

One of these substances is called lauric acid. This is well known as an antimicrobial agent. Microbes on the scalp have been identified as one reason that hair may be lost from the scalp. The microbes may collect in hair follicles and cause weakened low quality hair to be produced. Lauric acid can help prevent the build up of these microbes in hair follicles. This then, in turn, helps to stimulate new growth, which is also stronger and healthier. Lauric acid seems to be particularly good at stimulating new growth at and around the hair line. The substance called capric acid is another antimicrobial agent which is found in coconut oil and acts in a similar way to lauric acid. The antimicrobial action of coconut oil protects against scalp infections and dandruff as well as preventing hair follicle infections. All of this leads to better quality hair and less of the hair falling out due to weakness.

To deal with dandruff you should use a circular motion to massage the oil into the scalp. This will help to remove the scales of dead skin cells that characterize the dandruff condition. This massaging will also moisturize the skin layers below the surface of the scalp, which will help to prevent future occurrences of dandruff. The lauric acid will use its antimicrobial nature to kill any bacteria and fungi that could go on to cause dandruff at a later date. Regular use of coconut oil helps stop dandruff forming in a far gentler way compared to commercial anti dandruff shampoos. Coconut oil also contains vitamin E which is well known as being responsible for maintaining the health of the scalp skin. This vitamin maintains healthy hair production and helps to keep your hair shiny and bouncy.

A lot of people are gradually changing their usual hair care products for ones that use coconut oil as the main active ingredient. They are then reaping the benefits of this super conditioner. There is also a move to use coconut oil products for styling the hair as well. The reason for this is that the oil can be made to act in the same way as hair waxes and gels. In doing this job they moisturize the hair and scalp at the same time. Coconut styling products don't damage the hair in the same way that other styling products can. One key factor in the use of coconut oil in this area is the fact that it can keep moisturizing the hair at just about any temperature that is used during the styling process.

Treating head lice

Head lice attach themselves to the shaft of hairs and lay eggs which are referred to as nits. To treat head lice you have to get rid of both the live lice and the nits. Fine nit combs can be used to remove the nits but the live nits are difficult because of the way that they cling to the hairs.

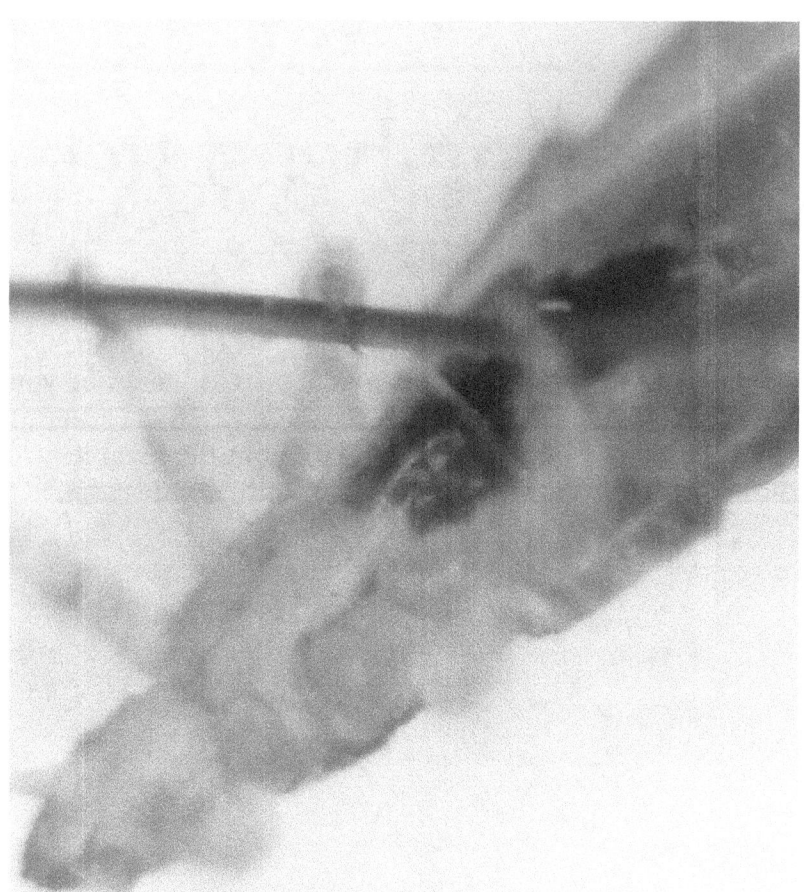

Head louse attached to a human hair

Coconut oil can be used in the control and eradication of head lice. You have to use a number of treatments with the coconut oil to successfully remove them. Firstly, to get rid of the visible lice in the hair take about five ml of coconut oil and warm it up so that it has melted. Apply the oil to the hair just before bedtime and massage it into the roots. Put a towel on the pillow to collect any of the dead or dying lice. The next morning shampoo the hair to help remove the dead lice. By this time the lice should have suffocated and will be easy to remove. The nits will also have swollen up with the oil and have become soggy and soft. After this you have to perform follow up treatments every two or three days to ensure that any newly hatched lice are removed. Lice have a seventeen day incubation cycle, so in order to get rid of them you need to keep doing the follow up treatments for up to around three weeks. Follow up treatments involve parting the hair down the middle and applying a few drops of coconut oil down the parting line and then above each of the ears. Throughout the day the oil will spread throughout the hair and will kill any of the newly hatched lice. The easiest way to apply the oil is to dip your finger in the oil and then just dab it onto the scalp where you need to put it.

Caring for your skin with coconut oil

As with the scalp, the rest of your skin will benefit from the use of coconut oil. For a start, the vitamin E in coconut oil will help to keep your skin healthy and young looking. It will help stop spots forming and help protect it from skin cancer. The antioxidant nature of vitamin E means that it will help deal with free radicals formed in the skin due to the body's exposure to smoke, ultraviolet light and pollutants. This can also help to enhance the working of any sun screens that you are using when on holiday in hot countries. The vitamin E content can also be beneficial in preventing the effects of aging such as wrinkles, age spots and stretch marks.

As mentioned with the hair, coconut oil also acts as a super moisturizer. You can therefore use it all over your body moisturizing every little bit of your skin. This totally natural product is unlikely to cause any adverse reactions such as rashes even on the most sensitive parts of the skin. This fantastic moisturizer will cost you the fraction of expensive petroleum based ones and will last a long, long time

As well as moisturizing, the active ingredients in coconut oil can have beneficial effects on certain skin conditions such as eczema, dermatitis and psoriasis. Tribute to this fact is that coconut oil is added to many skin treatments for these conditions all across the world.

In terms of skin infections, which can result is spots and inflammation, not only does the vitamin E do its magic job but added to this you have the anti microbial effects of the lauric acid and capric acid mentioned earlier. With all these ingredients acting together the skin is maintained in tip top condition.

You need the best organic cold pressed coconut oil for your own personal skin care. If you are using a lot of different products, and still getting nowhere with your skin care, especially if it is very dry then you should be able to dispense with everything else and concentrate on just using the coconut oil. Make sure that your coconut oil is in a glass container. You certainly don't want coconut oil that has been sitting in plastic containers. The reason for this is that chemicals from within the plastic can enter the coconut oil and this will reduce its effectiveness. You can use a little of the coconut oil on your finger to moisturize your lips. This is especially good for in the winter time. In winter the skin tends to get a lot drier due to the effects of the cold weather. At this time you should take just a very small amount of the coconut oil on your fingers and dab it over your face and just let it rest there for a while. If you find that you have put too much oil on your face simply take a clean towel and lightly tap the towel over your face. This will then remove the excess coconut oil.

The face is obviously the most important to concentrate on because it is so exposed to the elements, however, you can use the coconut oil on the skin all over your body. The most important thing is to use just a little of the oil. The longer that you use coconut oil on your skin the less frequently you will need to apply it because the moisture is retained in the skin by the oil. Coconut has a healing effect so you should notice that pimples and other infections will start to disappear.

Coconut oil can be used as part of your makeup routine. An example of this is where you can use the oil as a makeup remover. Simply rub over the make up and then rinse it way. When removing mascara from the eyes, once again apply the coconut oil, rinse away and then apply some fresh coconut oil to act as an eye cream. This eye cream with all of its vitamin E and antioxidants now also acts as an anti wrinkle cream.

When shaving, coconut oil can be used as a moisturizer both before and after shaving. This will give a clean shave that is really gentle on your skin. As well as this coconut oil won't clog the pores in the skin either.

Coconut oil can be used as an effective burn treatment. Apply the coconut oil generously to the burn area. It will have a cooling effect which will help to remove the pain from the burn. Coconut oil will give such good moisturizing that skin will remain very supple. This means that it will help to stop any blistering peeling or scarring in the area of skin that got burnt. The antimicrobial action will keep infections at bay and healing will be quicker.

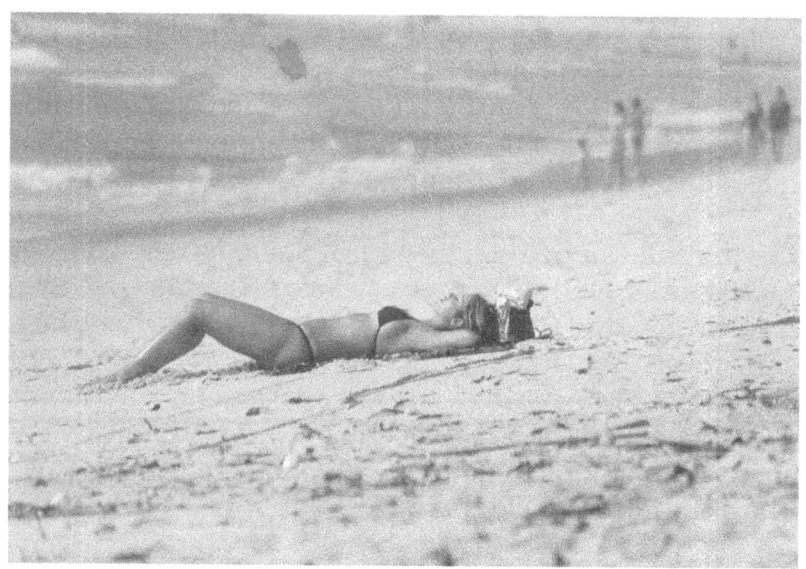

Coconut oil can be used as a sunscreen

Sunburn is another area where coconut oil can be of great use. Apply the coconut oil after showering. It will act like an after sun lotion, but will be more effective. The coconut oil will soothe the burning sensation, reduce the redness and will speed up the healing process within the skin. Repeat the application each day after showering and you will have super soft skin with no peeling. However, there is no need to end up with sunburn, in the first place, because coconut oil can be used as an effective sunscreen. Polynesian peoples have been using coconut oil as a sunscreen for thousands of years. It is a part of their tradition. Before going out to work for the day they apply a thin layer of coconut oil to their skin to protect themselves from the sun's rays. The coconut oil also tones up the skin and has the added advantage of keeping insects at bay as well. If you apply coconut oil to your own skin before going out into the sun it will protect you from burning.

The coconut oil acts as a sunscreen preventing the ultra violet light responsible for sunburn getting through to your skin. As well as this, the antioxidants and vitamin E in coconut oil help to prevent any damage to the skin occurring. It is no surprise therefore that the first sun lotions that were made in the Western world used coconut oil as one of their main ingredients. Modern sunscreens, of course, contain many other chemical ingredients so, if you want to avoid these, the best thing to do is to go back to basics and use pure raw coconut oil instead. After all, thousands of years of product testing can't be wrong! Pure coconut oil is easy to use on the skin as it soaks in almost immediately and doesn't leave a greasy residue to annoy you.

Coconut oil can also be used as massage oil. If you work with computers you can rub a small amount onto your shoulders for a few minutes and this will take the away any stress that you have built up while working. This will then allow you to be more focused on the work that you have to do. You can also use it as an all over body massage oil. The delightful feel and smell of the oil make it a very enjoyable experience, Coconut oil is edible so it can be a very interesting massage oil for couples to use in their relaxation time.

Mouth care with coconut oil

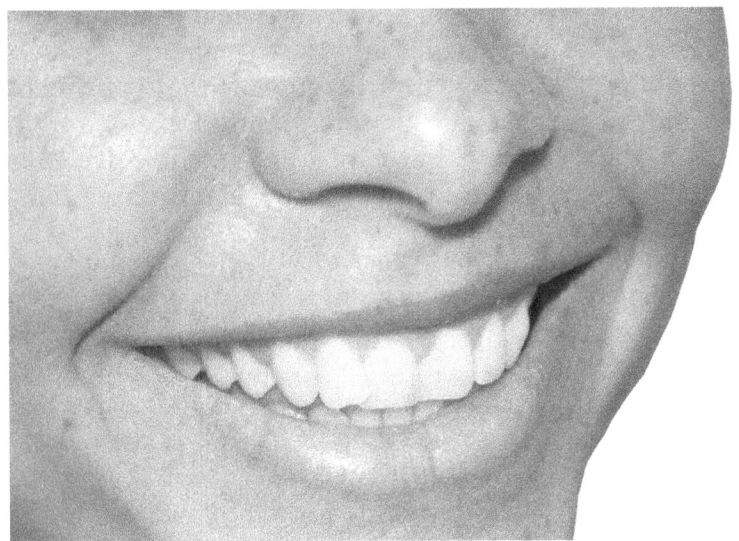

Use coconut oil on the gums and teeth

You can use coconut oil on sensitive areas of the gums. Just rubbing a little on these areas will allow it to deal with any infections. It also has a soothing action as well as tasting good. You should remember that the quality of your skin depends upon other factors such as diet and exercise. As a result you should make sure that you have a balanced diet and do regular exercise so that the coconut oil has a chance of doing a good job when you apply it to your skin.

Coconut oil can also be used as a method to whiten your teeth. In this case you need to take a spoonful of the oil and put it into your mouth and then swish it around in the same way that you would do with a mouth wash. Keep doing this for about ten or fifteen minutes. This is quite a long time to be doing this so make sure that you are doing something else such as taking a shower at the same time. This will take your mind off the coconut oil in your mouth and the time will soon pass by. After this time, you should spit all of the oil out and clean out any remains with fresh water. The antibacterial nature of coconut oil means that any infections or potential infections in the mouth are dealt with. This will also deal with any plaque bacteria that are on the teeth as well, which means that your teeth will remain white instead of becoming discolored due to the action of the bacteria in the plaque. Results with your mouth and teeth should be seen within days. This technique of improving mouth hygiene is referred to as 'Oil Pulling' which is an Ayurvedic healing and health tradition, which has been used for hundreds of years. The other benefits of this treatment include pinker looking and healthier gums as well as fresh breath. Ayurvedics say that oil pulling has further benefits for the whole of the body, however, one thing is for sure and that is that it certainly has a direct effect on mouth hygiene.

Acne control using coconut oil

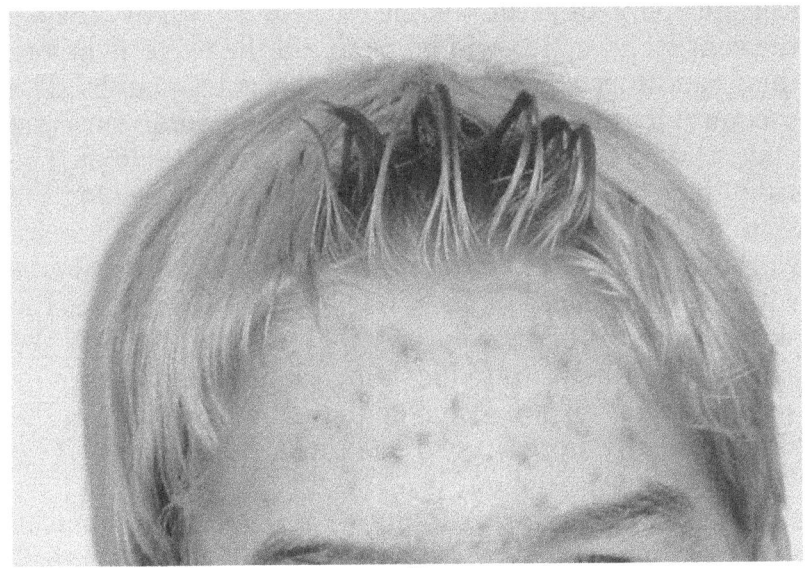

Use coconut oil to treat acne

Acne is a skin condition caused by the infection and blocking of sebaceous glands. These glands produce an oily substance called sebum which helps to keep the skin in good condition. Once they become blocked, due to infection by bacteria, the area of skin around the gland becomes red and inflamed and this is what we see on the surface of the skin and refer to as acne.

Usually the skin is able to maintain its resistance to infection because of the actions of friendly bacteria on its surface. The friendly bacteria release substances similar to the lauric acid in coconut oil. If the skin conditions change and the good bacteria no longer thrive, this is when infections of the sebaceous glands can occur. It is for this reason that acne is a lot worse amongst teenagers. Hormonal changes in the body at this age cause the skin to become a lot greasier with a lower pH and the friendly useful bacteria find it more difficult to thrive.

Coconut oil is of great benefit for acne sufferers because the capric and lauric acid helps to kill the bacteria before they can infect and block the sebaceous glands. The coconut oil can be applied directly to the skin or the same effect can be seen when it is taken as part of the diet. The vitamin E in coconut oil also plays its part by keeping the skin healthy and ensuring that the sebaceous glands are working, in good order and not blocked. This then helps with the exact cause of acne. Coconut oil also soothes the skin. It is absorbed easily and then soaks deep into the skin where it helps to reduce the inflammation caused by acne. Coconut oil will also help to heal any wounds in the skin caused by more aggressive forms of acne.

Another good effect of coconut oil is achieved by the way that it stabilizes the metabolic rate of the body. This then improves the quality of sebum secretions from the sebaceous glands as well as helping to correct any hormonal imbalances. If you suffer from acne, it is well worth giving coconut oil a try. Obviously, as with any treatment, results will vary from one individual to another, but if this works for you then you will have clearer skin and a healthier bank balance compared to those using other different trendy treatments advertised on our TV screens.

The trick with using coconut oil in the treatment of acne is to only use a little of it at a time. If you use too much it will block the pores and increase your problems. When you first start using coconut oil it will tend to make it worse initially and you need to prepare for this. You need to persist with the treatment despite this, and as time goes by the oil will help to clean out all of the pores and it will also deeply moisturize the skin. The antimicrobial nature of the coconut oil will kill any infective agents on the skin and the acne will start to get better. Coconut oil is not an actual cure for acne but rather a way of keeping it under control.

Coconut oil for weight loss

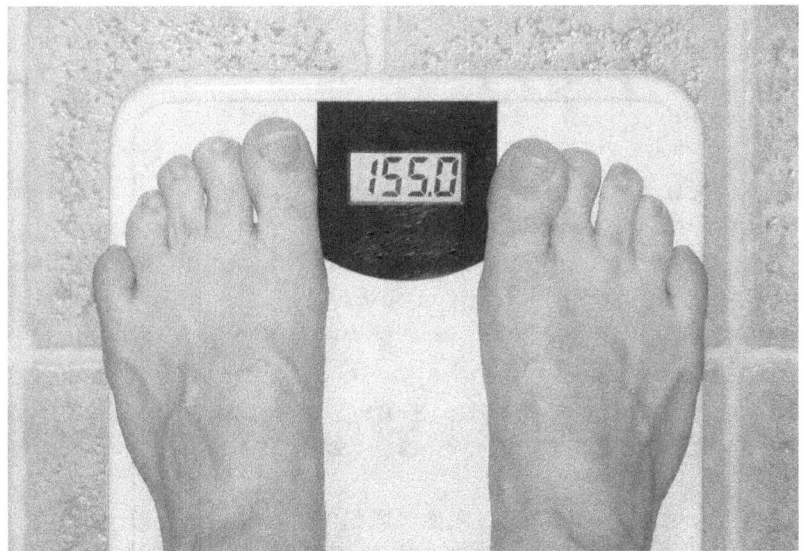

Shed the pounds with coconut oil

It seems ridiculous to suggest that eating a food which is high in fat content is going to help you reduce your weight. However, in the case of coconut oil this is just the situation! In fact ninety percent of coconut oil is made up of saturated fats. This seems to go against all that we have been told about fats and in particular saturated fats. We are told that even thinking about eating this type of fat will pile on the pounds. Indeed, eating saturated fats from sources such as butter, fatty meat and lard will quickly add to your weighty problem. The key to this anomaly centers on the kinds of saturated fats involved.

Not all saturated fats are built the same and as a result they don't all have the same effects on the human body. The saturated fats originating from meat and dairy products enter the blood stream after being processed in the digestive system and are then either broken down for energy in the liver or stored as fatty tissues around organs and under the skin as storage products. If glucose is also available, then this will be used to produce energy rather than the fats. The more fats that are consumed, the more of these that have to be stored for later use. It is this storage of excess fats that leads to people becoming overweight.

Most people trying to lose weight therefore have to try and get these stored fats to be used up by the body. There are 2 ways of achieving this. The first method involves taking in less food than you need each day. This then leads to the stored fat having to be used to provide energy for the body. The other way is to do a lot of exercise and this too can lead to the stored fats being used up to provide the extra energy that the body needs.

Diets usually use a combination of these methods to achieve their results. So as a result we are told to eat less and exercise more. The problems with these types of diet are that firstly the body automatically reduces its need for energy and secondly the body craves for the food that it is missing. The end result of these 2 effects is that people end up on a dieting plateau where they can't lose any more weight and cravings for food lead to people quitting their diets because they are too difficult to endure over long periods of time. Even people who actually lose weight on a diet plan aren't free from problems because once they are off their diet they quickly start consuming more food, and with the body working with lower energy needs the weight may be quickly put back on.

In the case of coconut oil the situation is very different because the saturated fats in it behave in a completely different way. Normal fatty acids from meat and dairy fats are hard for the body to break down and as a result are often just stored away. In contrast to this the fats from coconut oil are more easily broken down. The digestion products are medium chain fatty acids and can be used almost immediately for energy. Therefore these fatty acids don't tend to get stored like the other ones and as a result they won't add to your weight problem.

In addition to this, lauric acid, which is one of the fatty acids found in coconut oil, has another property and that is to increase the rate of metabolism in the body. The thyroid which controls metabolism therefore works at its optimum level. This means that the body will burn off more energy rich foods from one day to the next. We all know of people who can't seem to get fat, no matter what they eat. The reason for this is often that they have a high metabolic rate. In contrast to this people who have a low metabolic rate will tend to get fat because energy rich foods are burnt off at a far slower rate. As a result the presence of lauric acid in the diet will mean that you will burn off food at a faster rate and it will even cause the body to slowly use up the fat reserves around your organs and under the skin. In other words you will start to lose weight.

The key to getting the most out of coconut oil and the lauric acid is to add it to your diet in relatively small amounts. After all, fifty percent of virgin coconut oil is made up of lauric acid containing compounds. As you can see the concentration of this fatty acid is high. The metabolic rate increasing effect of consuming virgin coconut oil can last up to twenty four hours after initially eating it. This means that it is best to consume coconut oil regularly to maintain the effect.

Probably the best and easiest way to supplement your diet with coconut oil is to use it instead of any vegetable oil that you would normally use in cooking. There are also foods such as curries and stir fries where coconut oil is really a more natural thing to use. You have to realize that where these dishes originate from, coconut oil would often have been used anyway. The use of other vegetable oils in these dishes is often due to a westernization of the original recipes. Another way to do this is to add coconut milk to the meals that you cook. This can be used to make foods such as curries creamier as well.

Another factor in the diet equation is how hungry that you feel when you are on a diet. Reduced fat diets often end up making people feel a lot hungrier in general. This will mean that they will tend to feel hungry between meals and there is a great temptation to snack. Overall, these feelings of hunger can be too much to keep under control and as a result a lot of people will quit their diet and return to their usual eating regime. The opposite is also true in that, if you have fat in your diet you are less likely to feel these hunger pangs. The fat tends to lie in the stomach and this will make you feel full for longer. You will be less likely to snack and less likely to quit your diet. Obviously this would be like walking a tightrope with a normal diet because the fats you consume to stop you feeling hungry will just end up adding to your weight problem when the body decides to store them. However, if you substitute the fats from coconut oil the situation is different. You get the appetite reducing effect of the fats in your stomach but these fats are then readily used up to provide energy and more of the stored fats are used up because of the higher metabolic rate created by the effect of the lauric acid in the coconut oil.

If you compare the fats in coconut oil to those in meat and dairy products you will find that they contain less energy stored per gram. This means that virgin coconut oil isn't as energy rich as normal saturated fats and potentially you can consume more of them. This would therefore appear to be a win, win situation, and it is, so long as you don't consume too much of the virgin coconut oil. You have to realize that even the fats in coconut oil contain a lot of stored energy. This is the reason that it is best to just substitute it for your usual vegetable oils rather than gulping down jars of the stuff as if it is a medicine! Coconut oil could therefore enhance the effects of any diet regime that you might choose, and it certainly could make being on a diet easier to stomach.

Research into the effectiveness of coconut oil in dieting was undertaken by the 2009 study by the Garvan Institute in Sydney Australia. Although their experiments were on mice rather than humans the results are a good indication of why we people say that coconut oil helps them to lose weight. The results back up other studies in humans where medium chain fatty acids included in diets seem to help in weight loss. In the research different groups of mice were given a diet based on coconut oil or lard fat. The lard diet is more like a standard Western diet which would have something like forty percent saturated fat, forty percent monounsaturated fat and twenty percent of polyunsaturated fats. In this kind of diet there are also a greater proportion of omega 6 fatty acids compared to omega 3. People who have a weight problem that you would consider to fall into the obese category would typically consume forty percent of their calorie intake as fat. In the mice experiment the fat intake was set at forty five percent. High fat diets aren't good for the body. In a Western style high fat diet it leads to an overload of fats which the body can't deal with. Therefore, this type of diet results in the obesity epidemic that we see in countries such as the USA.

The amount of fat stored in the tissues of the body depends upon how much fat is taken up by the cells and how much of it is then burnt up for its energy needs. The body's natural reaction is to try and deal with this by increasing its ability to use fat for its energy needs. The medium chain fatty acids from coconut oil were found to be better at inducing this change to fat metabolism when compared to the long chain fatty acids found in the lard based diet. This means that the coconut oil diet led to less fat being deposited in muscles and fatty tissues of the body. It is thought that the reason for this is that the medium chain fatty acids are small enough to directly enter the mitochondria power houses of the cells where they can then be burnt up to provide energy. This is what we would consider as an increase in fat metabolism. The larger lard type fatty acids need to be broken down first in order to get into the mitochondria. This is very interesting because it helps to explain why people eating the medium chain fatty acids from coconut oil can actually lose weight.

There is a problem concerned with consuming a lot of medium chain fatty acids, such as those in coconut oil and this is that it can lead to the build up of fat in the liver. This is an important factor which should definitely be taken into consideration by anybody thinking of taking up a coconut oil based diet to help them lose weight. However, it is thought that the addition of fish oils to the diet could deal with the liver fat problem. The reason for this is that fish oils have a lot of metabolic benefits including that of improving the use of fat in the liver itself. A summary of the Garvan Institute scientific paper can be found at the following URL:

http://www.garvan.org.au/news-events/news/how-coconut-oil-could-help-reduce-the-symptoms-of-type-2-diabetes.html

Coconut oil cures for digestion problems

Coconut oil has been used for centuries as a medicinal agent to help with both normal digestion and people who have digestive problems. Its addition to curries and a lot of Asian recipes helps to make these foods both very appetizing and easy to digest.

Virgin coconut oil has strong antimicrobial properties and this can be put to use in maintaining digestive systems. Many digestion conditions may be caused by the presence of microbes in the food that we eat. Coconut oil can help to control the actions of these bad microbes. At the same time coconut oil has also been shown to help the good natural microbes in the gut. These natural microbes help in the absorption of vitamins from the digestive system and therefore maintaining them in good condition can have far reaching benefits for the whole body.

Coconut oil can also help in the fight against indigestion. It can help to stop the acid in the natural digestive juices in the stomach attacking the stomach wall. By stopping the acids irritating the stomach wall such conditions as acid reflux and ulcers can be avoided.

It has also been suggested that coconut oil can help in the treatment of more severe digestive conditions such as

Crohn's disease and ulcerative colitis. These conditions can be very distressing for the people suffering from them. Crohn's disease is an inflammatory intestinal condition which results in diarrhea, bleeding ulcers, stomach pain, anemia, bloody feces and loss of weight. In addition to this, ulcers can occur at any place along the digestive tract. Ulcerative colitis is in some ways like Crohn's disease but affects the lower part of the intestine called the colon.

One of the main problems that sufferers of these conditions have to put up with is nutritional deficiencies because the absorption of digested food is disrupted. They also find that a number of foods will cause their condition to get worse and as a result they find it difficult to find foods that they can consume with ease. Coconut oil, in the form of cookies, has proved to be a valuable tool in providing much needed nutrition for people with these conditions. The Medium Chain Fatty acids in coconut oil are easily digested and absorbed from the gut. For these patients, with disorders of fat digestion, absorption and transport, coconut oil provides an ideal solution. In addition to this, the oil can be self administered which is a great bonus compared with the drugs used that have to be administered by a health professional.

There is also anecdotal evidence that patients having coconut oil get relief from the symptoms of the disease and that it prevents digestive stress. The properties of coconut oil include anti inflammatory and healing properties and it is thought that it is these that provide the help with these rather severe conditions. It is thought that these diseases may be initiated by certain types of bacteria and viruses, especially those associated with such things as measles. These bacteria and viruses bore into the wall of the stomach and the rest of the digestive system causing the open sores that we associate with ulcers. It is interesting to note that it has been shown that the MCFA in coconut oil can easily kill these micro organisms. Further research may provide a direct link between the relief of these conditions and the actions of coconut oil on microorganisms in the gut.

Older people can also benefit from coconut oil. This is because the digestive process slows down with age and organs like the pancreas fail to make the amounts of digestive juices that they once did when the body was young. In addition to this, the small intestine doesn't absorb digested food as well either. As a result the whole process moves at a much slower pace. This can then result in a lack of minerals and vitamins. This where coconut oil comes in: because it is easily digested and at the same time mineral absorption is improved.

In a similar way coconut oil can be used with the very young too. It is included in most infant formulae for this reason. The MCFA are absorbed more easily than other fats and they lead to direct energy production in the liver and other cells. This puts less stress on little bodies and gives them a better chance of survival if they have digestive problems.

Immunity and fighting against infections

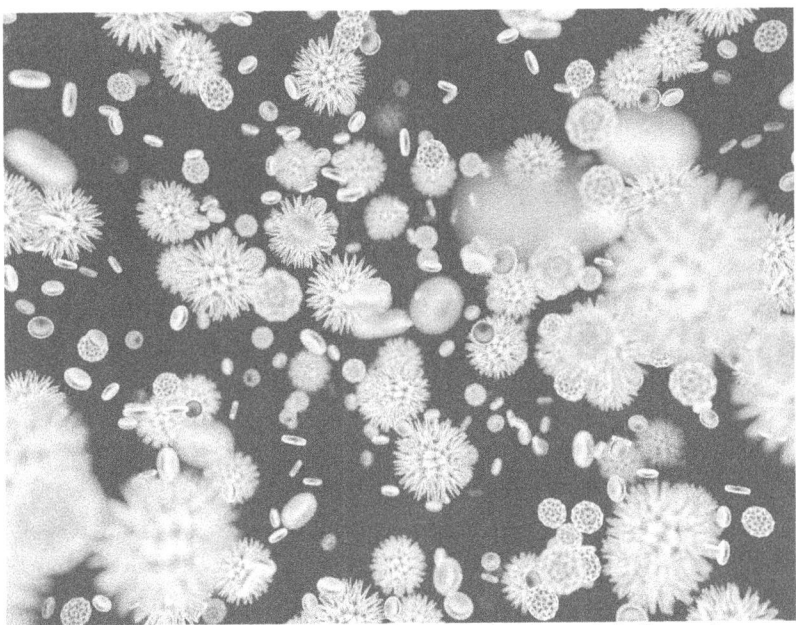

Coconut oil has a strong antimicrobial action

The immune system of the body relies on the production of antibodies which help destroy any invading pathogens such as bacteria, viruses, fungi and protozoan organisms. Normally the body is able to fight off these disease causing organisms, but there are occasions when it needs a helping hand. This is similar to the situation when you go to doctor and he prescribes antibiotics for an infection that doesn't want to go away. It would seem that coconut oil could also play a part in helping the body fight infection. This could become more important in the future because microorganisms such as bacteria are quickly learning how to get round the actions of our commonly used antibiotics. You only have to note the number of cases of hospital antibiotic resistant organisms such as MRSA.

One of the differences in the action of coconut oil compared to other antimicrobials is that rather than supplying a ready made antibacterial substance it provides the building blocks for the body to construct new antibacterial compounds. The active ingredient in coconut oil that has proved to be so important is lauric acid. The body uses this raw material to make a compound called monolaurin. This is the same anti microbial agent that babies produce from lauric acid provided in their mother's milk. Babies depend on this because their immune systems are far too immature to act on their own. This monolaurin stops infants from succumbing to bacterial, viral or protozoan based infections. Despite its link with fighting infection in infants this property of coconut oil hadn't really been taken seriously up until a few years ago.

It was first noted in the 1960s that particular fatty acids and the compounds produced from them had the property of deactivating a number of different microorganisms. These included bacteria, membrane enveloped viruses and fungi including yeasts.

Monolaurin acts on these organisms by disrupting the phosphor lipid membranes that surround them. It does this by making the membranes more soluble and as a result they start to disintegrate. In the case of viruses the envelope around them breaks down. Not all viruses are deactivated by maonolaurin as it depends upon their individual structure. However, there are a number of important pathogenic viruses that are deactivated such as HIV, herpes, VSV, visna virus and Cytomegalovirus. On top of this, there are many opportunistic disease causing organisms that are also disrupted by monolarin. These are the same kind of organisms that cause infections in HIV positive people. As a result coconut oil could become an important dietary addition for people infected with HIV as it is the secondary infections that cause so many problems for these individuals. It is important to note that these fatty acids and compounds derived from coconut oil are not toxic to human cells despite their effect on such a range of microorganisms. This is because they are essentially produced by human cells themselves from the raw ingredients in the coconut oil. Monolaurin derived from coconut oil has been described as one of the best inactivating fatty acid derived substance that is currently known.

Coconut oil can also be applied externally to deal directly with a range of infections. It is very good for treating cuts, scrapes and bruises. Once applied to the affected area the coconut oil keeps it free from infection. In addition to this the moisturizing property of the oil helps the skin to heal by providing the nutrients and conditions needed for the repair of the skin tissue. There is also an observed effect of tightening the skin which seems to help prevent stretch marks and bad scarring from an injury.

Fight off Candida with coconut oil

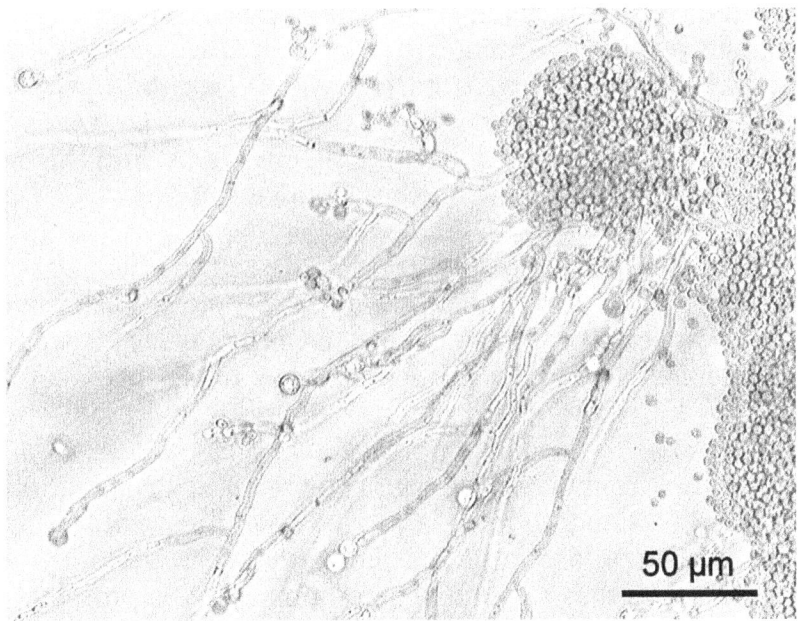

Candida fungi under the microscope courtesy of Y tambe

Candida is a yeast infection that is often wrongly diagnosed or simply dismissed as nothing of any importance. Despite this it is often found to be behind many other visible health problems such as chronic tiredness, memory problems, bad mood swings, sinus infections and coughs, blurred vision and even cravings for sugary foods. People have also described many other symptoms relating to yeast infections of this kind. It is estimated that up to forty million people in the USA may be suffering from Candida with many of them simply not realizing what is going on within their bodies. These people end up trying to treat the symptoms without dealing with the main issue and this may continue on for many years before a correct diagnosis is forth coming. The problems don't stop their either: because even if the find the root cause of their problems they will often be let down by the usual drugs that are on offer to treat Candida. In addition to this the drugs used can have many side effects which can end up being worse than the yeast infection that they started with. As a result, people in this situation are always looking for alternative treatments to try and alleviate their problems, and this is where coconut oil can come into its own.

Coconut oil is an effective treatment for fungi and yeast infections such as candida. Candida can affect both men and women but women seem to have the most persistent problems. Infections can include areas of the body such as the digestive system, genitalia, mouth and scalp. A number of women have found that candida can be prevented from occurring simply by including coconut oil in the diet. Candida itself is usually kept under control by friendly bacteria on the skin however, when the body is under stress these friendly bacteria may not be promoted and that is when candida and other yeast infections can take a hold. Capric acid is the main ingredient in coconut oil which seems to be most effective against candida.

Coconut oil is also gentle on the skin and can be used by people who have adverse reactions to other stronger anti fungal drugs. It is interesting to note that in areas of the world where coconuts are grown extensively and make up a high proportion of the local diet women are rarely affected by these types of yeast infections. With as many

62

as 40 million people suffering with candida there is a need for an easy self administered non toxic treatment such as that provided by coconut oil. Candida is one of those conditions which can keep recurring and for this reason it is a good idea to maintain coconut oil in your diet rather than just using it when the yeast infection symptoms occur.

To use coconut oil internally to fight Candida you should take about 3 tablespoons of the oil each day in your diet. If you haven't taken coconut oil before you should start off with about a teaspoon of the oil each day and slowly work up to the full 3 tablespoon dose. The worse that you have the condition, then the more slowly that you should work towards the full dose. The reason for this is because the yeast fungus can die off really quickly and this can cause the body to react against it. The symptoms of this are often flu like with chills, headache and tiredness. This may last up to a weak depending on how severe the Candida actually is. The best thing to do is to slowly increase the amount of coconut oil that you take so that this sudden die off doesn't occur.

You can also use coconut oil directly on some visible fungal infections. Simply apply a small amount of the coconut oil to the affected area three or four times per day. This treatment is suitable for such things as athlete's foot, jock itch or yeast rash. This local treatment will be more effective if you are also taking coconut oil as part of your diet. If 3 tablespoons of coconut oil seems to be a lot then you can try taking it in different ways such as using it instead of butter when you make toast, adding it to coffee or tea and mixing it with oatmeal when you make porridge.

Coconut oil and type 2 diabetes

Type 2 diabetes is gaining epidemic proportions. In the USA the numbers of people becoming diabetic is doubling every ten years. It is a huge problem with over eight percent of the US population having the condition. As usual, the pharmaceutical companies are cashing in on this record number of sufferers. The problem is that the drugs that they develop deal with the symptoms of the condition rather than the actual cause of it. This means that people are forced to just get on with suffering and taking more medicines rather than getting a real cure. In addition to this, all of the drugs that are available have side effects which often stop people getting on with their normal lives.

It is now recognized that type 2 diabetes especially in the early stages is reversible. It is all about diet. The main problem is the amount of refined sugars that people are consuming. These refined sugars are responsible for the body becoming resistant to insulin. If you cut them out the resistance to insulin disappears and it is back to normal life. Weight also has an effect in diabetes as well, so dieting and exercise are also important. Loss of weight puts less stress on the body. All the cells in the extra body weight have to be maintained and it is this that puts the stress on the body that can result in insulin resistance. Changing your diet is, however, the important thing.

One of the problems with dieting is that people get cravings for these refined sugars and therefore it is difficult to maintain a diet and get back to your correct weight. The addition of coconut oil to your diet can cut down on the cravings for these refined sugars allowing you to maintain your diet and reach the weight that you need as well as reducing the same sugars responsible for the insulin resistance.

A lot of evidence about the effectiveness of coconut oil in the prevention of diabetes has been collected by the use of population statistics in countries such as India and the Polynesian islands in the Pacific Ocean. In these areas consuming coconut oil is a matter of tradition. It is found that within the population of coconut oil consumers diabetes is a very rare condition. This in itself is very good news, but in addition to this there is the opportunity to study other populations where they have abandoned their traditional coconut consumption in favor of polyunsaturated fats, such as that from sunflower seeds, and other processed foods. In these populations the amount of diabetes increases to the same levels as seen in the Western world.

Direct evidence of how coconut oil can be helpful in the case of diabetes can be seen in the case of the 2009 study by the Garvan Institute in Sydney Australia. This research was published in the international journal 'Diabetes'. Here a study on animals found that a diet with a lot of coconut oil protected against insulin resistance in the animal's cells. As well as this the coconut oil diet didn't cause an increase in body fat. The actual experiment involved feeding different diets to 2 groups of mice. They had either a diet rich in coconut oil or a diet rich in lard. The lard was to represent a typical Western diet. The results of this research are important because obesity and insulin resistance are the 2 major factors in determining if somebody will become diabetic. A summary of the Garvan Institute scientific paper can be found at:

http://www.garvan.org.au/news-events/news/how-coconut-oil-could-help-reduce-the-symptoms-of-type-2-diabetes.html

A study from 2010 in the Indian Journal of pharmacology studied the effects of fat diet on the fat profile of rats. They used diabetic and normal rats and fed them with a coconut rich diet for 45 days or a diet based on ground nut oil for the same amount of time. When they compared the results they found that the rats fed coconut oil had a greater tolerance to glucose compared with those fed on the ground nut oil based diet. This is thought to be caused by the larger amounts of lauric acid in the coconut oil. This tolerance to glucose is due to an increase in the cells sensitivity to insulin. This basically means that coconut oil improves the ability of body cells to deal with the excess glucose involved in type 2 diabetes. As well as this it was also found that the coconut oil rats had an improved fat profile in their body fluids and this resulted in less fat being laid down in arteries. Diabetics have a problem with fat build up in arteries and therefore need their fat profile assessed on a regular basis. It appears that coconut oil could help to maintain a healthy body fluid fat profile in diabetics. The study can be found on the internet at the following URL:

http://www.ncbi.nlm.nih.gov/pmc/articles/PMC2937313

Scientists and drug companies are now seriously interested in coconut oil as far as controlling diabetes is concerned. Obviously they can't patent coconut oil itself, but the rush is now on to try and find an active ingredient within coconut oil that they can then synthesize chemically and use in their drugs. At the moment they are concentrating on one of the fatty acids with this in mind. The particular medium chain fatty acid being focused on is capric acid. Scientific studies on this have revealed that it can help to control blood sugar levels.

Coconut oil to prevent heart disease

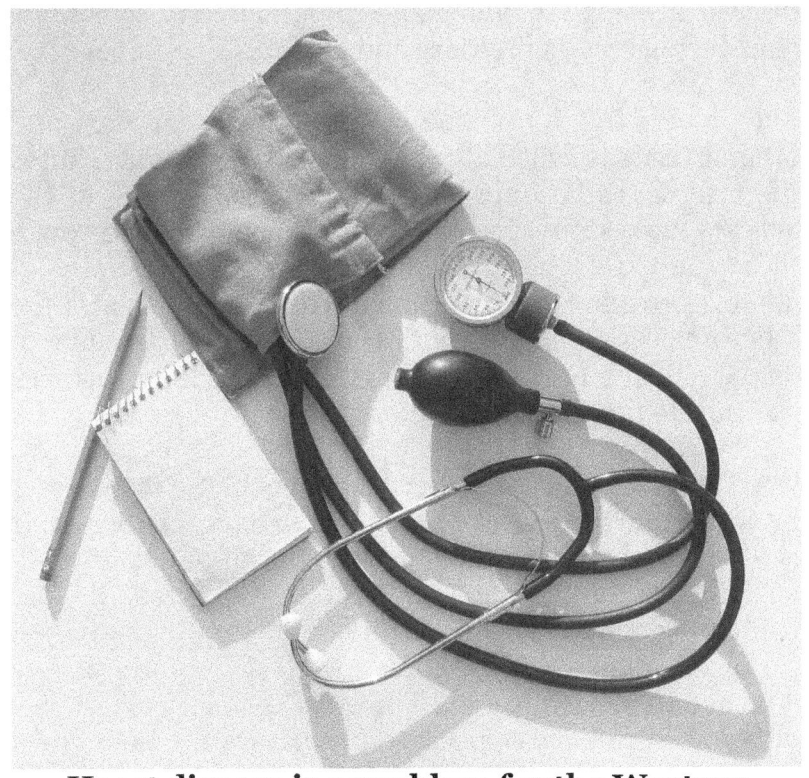

Heart disease is a problem for the Western World

Across the world heart disease is a major concern. It is responsible for more than 13 million deaths every year and in America more than 70 million people suffer from some sort of heart or circulatory problem. Out of all of the forms of cardiovascular disease the most common is coronary artery disease. This is caused by the build up of fatty plaque material in the small coronary artery which supplies oxygen and food to the heart muscles themselves.

The onset of coronary heart disease is mainly influenced by lifestyle choices and also by inherited characteristics. The main factors which can lead to coronary heart disease are high blood cholesterol, heredity, smoking, obesity, high blood pressure and diabetes.

The process of fatty plaque build up in the coronary and other arteries is called atherosclerosis. This in turn causes the arteries to become hardened. The hardening of the arteries makes it more difficult for blood to flow through them and this can in turn increase the rate of atherosclerosis. It is not known what actually starts the atherosclerosis process but it may initially be due to damage to the artery wall caused by such things as free radicals, toxins, bacteria and or viruses.

Once the damage has occurred platelets in the blood react by sticking to the damaged area in an attempt to heal it. It is at this point that other materials such as cholesterol, triglycerides and calcium become deposited in the damaged area. This leads to the build up of scar tissue. All of these materials become a part of the fatty plaque attached to the artery wall. The build up restricts the flow of blood in the artery because it narrows the hole down which the blood flows. This is doubly problematic in the small coronary arteries supplying the heart itself. The narrowing of the coronary artery also causes red blood cells to drag against the rough scar tissue. This can result in the increased risk of blood clots forming. This then, is coronary heart disease and a real killer in our modern world.

Saturated fats and trans saturated fats are responsible for the majority of the fats deposited in the atherosclerosis. This is because they lead to the build up of the bad LDL variety of cholesterol in the blood. This is the fatty stuff that gets deposited on the artery walls. It would therefore seem strange to recommend a type of saturated fat as a solution for the atherosclerosis problem, but this is just the case when considering coconut oil. Ninety percent of the oil is in a saturated form. This is one reason that coconut oil hasn't been taken seriously over the years.

In order to understand the importance of coconut oil you have to appreciate that the saturated fats in coconut are made up differently. Once again the Medium Chain Triglycerides come into play. As we have found out, these behave differently. These are broken down efficiently and then taken to the liver where they are burnt to provide energy. The usual long chain triglycerides from meat and dairy products aren't broken down like this and end up being repackaged in the liver as fatty proteins. These then have a bad effect on the level of LDL or bad cholesterol in the blood which in turn leads to atherosclerosis. Coconut oil has the opposite effect in that it increases the levels of the good HDL cholesterol. This type of cholesterol helps to protect the arteries against fatty build ups and in turn fights against heart disease.

It is well known that places like Sri Lanka and India have a very low incidence of coronary heart disease and this is now put down to the regular use of coconut oil in their cooking. It is also interesting to note that India is now having increasing problems with heart disease and this is since traditional coconut oil has been replaced by western style vegetable oils. The same situation has been seen where peoples from the Polynesian islands moved to New Zealand. The Polynesians had very little incidence of heart disease and used a lot of coconut oil as it is native to the islands. Once the people moved to New Zealand they started using vegetable oils instead and since then the incidence of heart disease in the migrated populations has rocketed.

Clearly it is obvious that despite the initial appearance of coconut as a bad oil containing bad saturated fats it is actually a better choice to other oils and should be used as often as possible in order to improve your diet and reduce the chance of heart disease.

Alzheimer's and dementia treatment

The fear of Alzheimer's amongst Western populations is only topped by the fear of getting cancer. This fear is also getting bigger as life span is increasing and the population of pensioners is getting larger. It is a horrible disease involving a person slowly having failing memory, strange behaviors and loss of normal body functions. I had to watch while my mother slowly withered and died away over a period of 6 years. I don't think that I have fully recovered from those lost years yet. It is no wonder that people will try almost anything to try and avoid the condition.

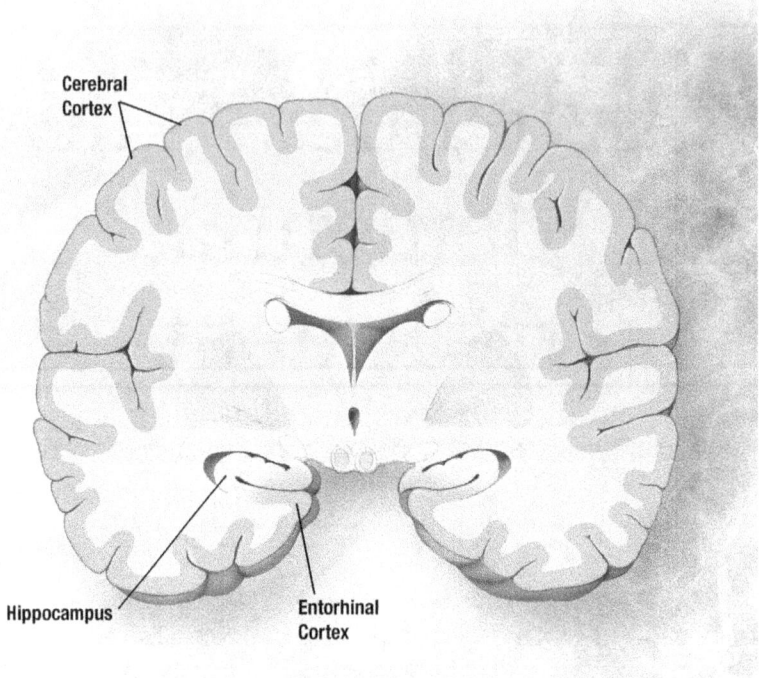

Labels on image: Cerebral Cortex, Hippocampus, Entorhinal Cortex

Normal brain cross section

There has been a lot of research into Alzheimer's but as yet there is no identifiable cure on the horizon. There have been the occasional revelation about a discovery but real results quickly fade into the distance as people fail to respond to proposed treatments. There are drugs which can delay the onset of the disease but as I discovered with my mother's case they can often have side effects that are far worse than the condition itself. The gains she made from the drug were very modest indeed and the doctors said that she may have gained 6 months and that was about it. Eventually she had to go into a home and have 24 hour care. At this point she had been robbed of real speech, concentration and even the ability to stand up. Even from here there was just over a year of undignified care until she eventually went to her maker. Some people have discovered that coconut oil can help them with this condition and this has led to scientific research into why this should be so.

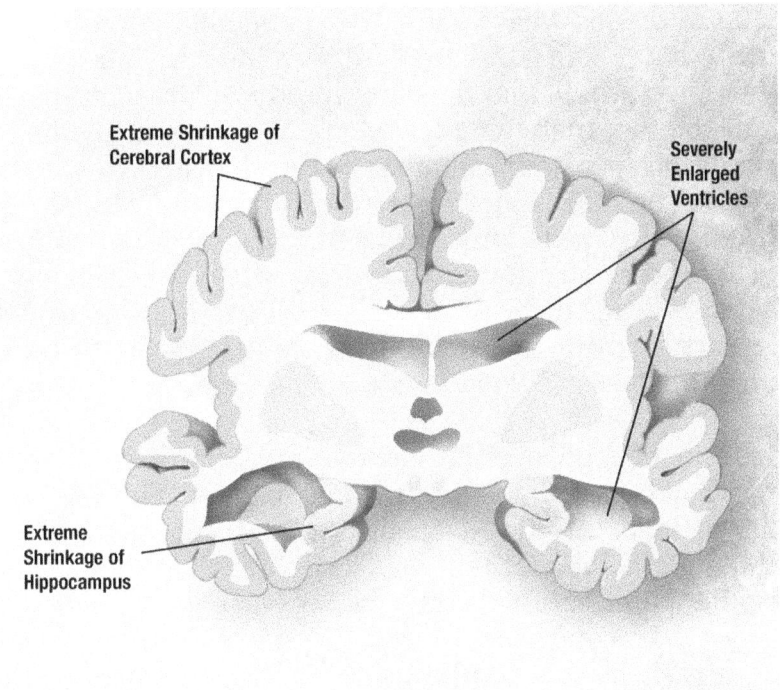

Extreme Shrinkage of
Cerebral Cortex

Severely
Enlarged
Ventricles

Extreme
Shrinkage of
Hippocampus

Alzheimer's brain cross section

The Alzheimer's condition in characterized by the development of plaques of the protein amyloid-β(Aβ) inside the brain. . It is thought that these plaques somehow prevent nervous connections happening within the brain. This then leads to the disruption of thoughts and memories that is seen in people suffering from Alzheimer's. Researchers have concentrated on these plaques in the search for a cure for the disease. The simple idea is that if you remove the plaques then the brain will regain its ability to communicate and that the thought process and memories will return. Most of the drugs that have been proposed and tested are designed to interfere in some way with the production of the amyloid-β(Aβ) protein. This should result in the delaying of the onset of the Alzheimer's condition. It is unfortunate that a lot of the tests have had to be abandoned when human trials have started. This has been due to a range of unrelated effects that the newly produced drugs have had and the fact that some have even made the Alzheimer's condition worse in a number of the subjects. This is the area where the majority of research money is and has been spent. The failures in this have led other researchers to propose a different idea about how Alzheimer's actually develops. This new research has been prompted in part from the anecdotal evidence that coconut oil can improve the condition of Alzheimer's sufferers.

Instead of studying the amyloid-β(Aβ) protein plaques which occur in the later stages of Alzheimer's they were determined to look at changes that occur in the early stages. It is thought that any observations at these times would point more directly to the actual cause of the disease. It may in fact be that the amyloid-β(Aβ) protein is merely the end result of a lot of other changes in the brain. Initial research into the early stages of Alzheimer's has found some interesting factors that are now being studied in more detail. It has been identified that there is a link between people who have a resistance to insulin and the onset of Alzheimer's. This has lead to it being referred to as a form of diabetes. In a small number of cases it has been found that the early stages of Alzheimer's is also linked to a problem inside cells themselves. Every cell has special organelles called mitochondria. These are the powerhouses of the cell and produce energy from glucose sugars. In Alzheimer's suffers the mitochondria don't function very well and as a result there isn't enough energy produced for the cell's needs. It also leads to the production of oxidizing compounds which can damage cells. When these cells are in the brain you can see that they won't be performing as well as they should and this in turn will restrict the mental ability of a person.

There has also been a lot of interest in dietary fat content and its effect on the brain. It should be noted that the majority of the brain is made up of fatty material. Amongst other things, the fat is used in the brain around nerve cells to insulate them from each other. This is a bit like the plastic cover around wires used in electrical circuits. Without this plastic insulation the electricity could easily move into other wires that it touches. In a similar way nerve cells need to transmit electrical signals down their length and the fatty sheaths around them stop any cross wires and also speed the signals along the length of the nerve cells. You should see that anything changing the fat content of the brain could easily affect its performance.

There is one particular type of fat that appears to be very important for brain function and that is cholesterol. There are 2 kinds of cholesterol. LDL cholesterol is low density and HDL cholesterol is high density cholesterol. The brain appears to need the LDL version of cholesterol for a healthy life. It has been found that people with high levels of LDL cholesterol in their blood tend to live longer and also have better mental acuity when they are older. It has also been suggested that the body will tend to increase the levels of blood cholesterol in an attempt to prevent Alzheimer's by increasing its availability to the brain. There is more and more evidence appearing which suggests that problems in the brain involving the use of cholesterol are responsible for the Alzheimer's condition. This has been backed up by the examination of the brain and spinal fluids. It has been found that in Alzheimer's sufferers the levels of cholesterol and triglycerides is much reduced. Cholesterol is also important for the integrity of the protective membrane around nerve cells.

With low LDL blood cholesterol the cell membranes are weaker which means that they are more prone to attack from bacteria and other pathogens as well as being more easily damaged by substances such as free radicals and hydrogen peroxide. This would all seem to suggest that brain health needs a good supply of LDL cholesterol from the blood stream. Population studies amongst the elderly have shown that those with brain conditions such as depression, Alzheimer's and Parkinson's have far lower blood cholesterol levels compared to those with out the conditions.

Alzheimer's probably starts with a problem in the supply of cholesterol and other fats to nerve cells in the brain. This then leads to damage due to oxidation and mitochondria that no longer work correctly. The nerve cells have to try and use other sources than glucose for producing their energy because they can no longer rely on their damaged mitochondria. Eventually the nerves can't transmit their electrical signals effectively. The cells produce amyloid-β(Aβ) as a substitute for cholesterol and to enable the cells to use alternative energy sources. The amyloid-β(Aβ) also helps to try and prevent oxidation damage to the cell's membrane. Eventually even the amyloid-β(Aβ) can not cope with the worsening situation within the nerve cell. At this point these cells are looked on as a danger to the rest of the healthy nerve cells around them and as a result they are destroyed by the body's own defense system. Destroyed cells mean lost memories and lost mental ability which are the classic symptoms of Alzheimer's sufferers.

The cell membranes of nerve cells in the brain need to be repaired all of the time. In order to do this they need to be provided with fresh supplies of LDL cholesterol. Unfortunately there has been a trend since the 1960s in making people have low cholesterol diets. This is mainly in response to another damaging condition which is heart

78

disease. Unfortunately LDL cholesterol has been targeted as the causative agent for this condition. People have not only been told to avoid cholesterol containing foods they have also been prescribed more and more cholesterol reducing drugs. In particular this has led to a large part of the drug industry being involved in the production of these heavily prescribed Statin type of medicines. We regularly get doctors saying that everybody over 50 should be given a pill to take every day to reduce the chance of getting heart disease. The main ingredient in these pills would be Statin based. This means that in the future the majority of people would be on cholesterol reducing drugs. It has however been noticed that as these low fat diets have taken hold and more and more Statins have been prescribed there has been a parallel increase in the numbers of people suffering from dementia. This is not direct proof that the two factors are related but it does give prevalence to the notion that the reduction in blood cholesterol levels in people could be linked to the problems that we are now seeing in more and more people's brains. More information about the proposed role of cholesterol depletion and Alzheimer's can be found by looking at the following research paper:

http://people.csail.mit.edu/seneff/EJIM_PUBLISHED.pdf.

This is a scientific paper published by the European Journal of Internal Medicine and as a result is very technical in its detail.

Due to the above indicated problems caused by the inability of brain cells to get the cholesterol that they require and the damage caused by oxidation it has been proposed that the best way to deal with Alzheimer's is to change your diet. The diet needs to have less processed carbohydrates and proportionally more fats and cholesterol. As well as this, the inclusion of antioxidants in the diet will also help to prevent the oxidative damage that is seen in Alzheimer's. This helps to explain how coconut oil can be good for Alzheimer's sufferers.

Medium Chain triglycerides in coconut oil seem to help with Alzheimer's. If you take 2 table spoons of virgin coconut oil every day you could see some positive results even within a day. The best way of taking this oil is with your cooking. However, you can make sure that you have the right amount by including it with your breakfast. You can add it to warm breakfast cereals such as oats. In this form it is also easier to eat because the warmth of the cereal tends to change the coconut oil into a more palatable liquid form.

People taking coconut oil for Alzheimer's have often described it as being like a light being suddenly turned on as their memory begins to be active once again. This does not mean that a person with this condition can expect a full recovery. There is a points system for determining the memory ability with Alzheimer's sufferers and it had been shown that people taking coconut oil could expect something like a 2 point increase in their ability on the scale used. This could be the difference in knowing where they are, the area where they live and other important information which allows people to be more independent in their day to day lives.

Although it isn't exactly clear how these increases in cognitive ability are actually achieved, it thought to be due to the way that Medium Chain Triglycerides are metabolized within the body. They are first delivered to the liver where they are broken down to form new compounds called ketone bodies. These are then released into the blood stream and travel around the body and in particular to the brain. Once in the brain it seems that the brain cells take up the ketone bodies more easily that the normal energy source of glucose. The damaged brain cells then use the ketone bodies to provide energy for the cells to do its work. The cells become more active and this often results in the return of short term memory ability. It is thought that reduced supply of energy rich compounds such as glucose to brain cells is responsible for a lot of the damage in the brain associated with the Alzheimer's condition. This lack of nutrients causes the brain cells to age before their time and then allows for the dementia condition to develop. In addition to providing an alternative energy source for brain cells it is also thought that coconut oil also has the effect of increasing the supply of blood to the brain and in doing so provides extra nutrients and oxygen for respiration. Ketone metabolism is the alternative energy source that the damaged cells need especially if the nerve cells have malfunctioning mitochondria and can't use glucose any more.

Coconut oil is not the total answer to dementia and as a result people should look at the rest of their diet, the amount of exercise they do and the level of mental stimulation that they get. It has been shown that taking exercise on a regular basis is a good way of preventing the occurrence of Alzheimer's. It is a well known fact that people in the Western world take less and less exercise the older that they get. This exercise can amount to walking for at least half an hour each day. In terms of mental stimulation it is a case of use your brain and memory or lose it. Certainly having coconut oil in your diet can help with Alzheimer's and it may also prevent people from getting the condition in the first place. Although coconut oil contains antioxidants it is best to have additional sources of these valuable compounds in your diet. Increasing the fruit content of your diet or consuming Rooibos tea is one way to increase your antioxidant intake. There is also the problem of the Statin drugs that people are taking for heart conditions. This is bound to reduce the effectiveness of the coconut oil that you consume. However, you should consult a medical professional about your Statin intake. You certainly shouldn't make any changes to the drugs that you take if they are prescribed by your doctor. However, if you think that these might be a problem you should discuss the amount that you are taking with the doctor that has prescribed them for you.

Anti cancer properties of coconut oil

Coconut oil has very strong anti cancer properties. This has been demonstrated in laboratory animal experiments where the animals were primed with chemicals to develop cancer. In one experiment all of the animals were given exactly the same diet apart from the type of oil included in it. Various oils were used including olive, corn and of course virgin coconut oil. The study involved determining the effect of these different oils on the prospect of developing colon cancer. It was found that all of the animals went on to develop cancer apart from those that had coconut oil in their diet. Coconut oil managed to block the development of colon cancer in these particular animals.

In another similar study researchers were investigating different oils on the development of breast cancer, and once again only those given coconut oil didn't get cancer. The researchers dissected the mammary glands of the animals but couldn't find any cancer in the rats on the coconut diet despite very strong cancer inducing chemicals being used.

In yet another study cancer causing chemicals were applied to the skin of animals and within a few weeks the tumors associated with skin cancer developed. However, if coconut oil was applied to the skin together with the chemicals it was found that the cancer didn't develop. There is even anecdotal evidence that people applying coconut oil to existing melanoma skin cancer areas have seen the cancerous tissue almost dissolve away over time. This is yet another reason for using coconut oil on your skin especially if you are going to be exposed to the sun.

Despite these encouraging animal studies there is, however, little evidence that coconut oil can prevent or cure cancer in humans according to science information officers at Cancer research UK. In general, research information is confusing as some studies show that coconut oil and other vegetable oils might have anti cancer properties, however, other studies have shown the exact opposite even up to the point that coconut oil might even promote cancer. It is clear that a lot more research is needed into coconut oil and cancer, but with so many other avenues of research into cancer it is unlikely that many studies will be carried out in this direction in the near future.

Conclusion

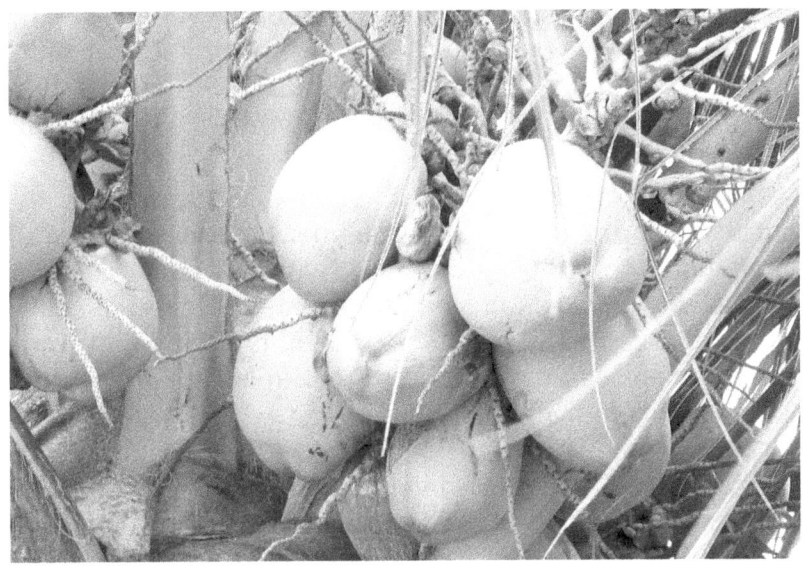

Once you start using coconut oil it is difficult to stop. We use it in the kitchen for the initial frying of such meals as Indian curries and Thai dishes. Once you have tasted the difference you wonder why you never used it before. I use it together with cocoa butter and Shea butter to make my own skin creams. The extra moisturizing effects of the coconut oil means that I no longer suffer from the bad eczema that I have had since being a child. Up until this point I had been using expensive treatments from a Chinese herbalist. It is far more effective and cheaper to just get a jar of coconut oil from the local health shop. My son also suffers from dry skin and I am now making a coconut oil based cream for his skin too.

I also make a hair conditioner with coconut oil as one of the ingredients. Coconut oil is ideal for making such things as leave in conditioners because it is so good for the scalp and hair. This hair conditioner has prevented the dandruff and dry patches on my scalp that I once suffered from. In addition to this I have found that hair that wouldn't grow at my hair line, due hair styling chemicals, has started to grow back. I am really impressed with how I have got into using coconut oil. I am now thinking of starting a business making skin creams because all of my friends have shown a great interest in buying them from me.

So, if you want to improve your health and the taste of your food you should definitely switch to using coconut oil instead of vegetable oil for cooking. Once you have gained the confidence of using this oil try using it on your skin. I am sure that you will be amazed at the difference it will make to your life.

There seem to be new and novel uses for coconut oil being discovered all of the time, for example: you can use coconut oil to remove chewing gum from your hair. This is achieved by rubbing some of the oil over the chewing gum and then leaving it for about half an hour before using your finger tips to roll the gum out of the hair. Another idea is that you can apply the coconut oil to your satellite dish to stop the snow sticking in the winter. How about using it as a lubricant on your electric guitar strings?

I have even found a new use for coconut oil in the last few days. I am using it to treat dandruff inside my ears. This is very itchy and annoying. I am applying just a thin smear of the coconut oil with my little finger to the inside of my ears. The itchy feeling disappears very quickly. A result at last!

There seem to be uses for coconut oil everywhere. Coconut oil really is a universal agent.

About the Author

Ellen Vincent has written a number of other books on alternative diets, foods and treatments based on natural ingredients. The first book gives the background as to why green smoothies are so healthy and how to make them. The second book details the health benefits of Apple cider vinegar. All books are published as paperbacks and on the kindle platform.

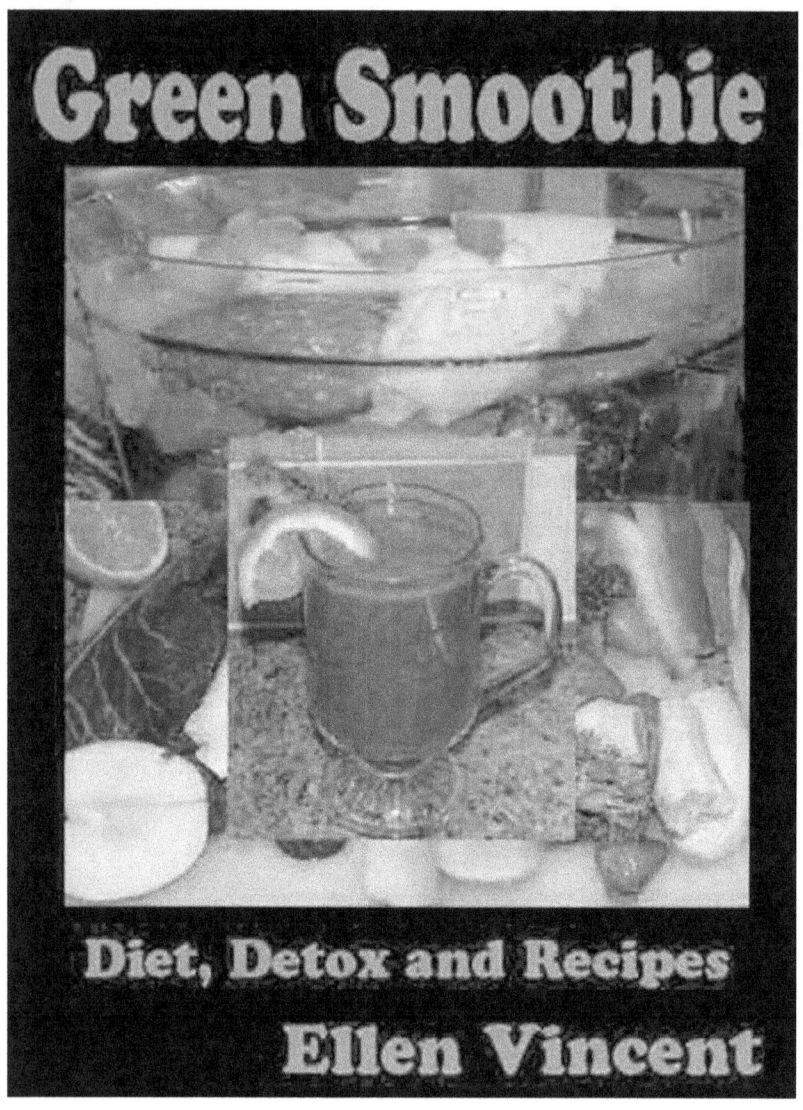

Kindle edition: http://www.amazon.com/Green-Smoothie-Detox-Recipes-ebook/dp/B007SP3K0C/

Paperback: http://www.amazon.com/Green-Smoothie-Diet-Detox-Recipes/dp/1475179731/

Green smoothies are very popular when it comes to dieting, detoxifying and giving the human body the nutrients that it needs in order to work at the peak of performance. This book explains the many ways that green smoothies can help your body and improve your health and life in general. There are plenty of tips on producing and tailoring green smoothies for your individual needs and there are over 100 exciting recipe ideas included in the book.

Green smoothies give you all of your nutrients the way that nature intended. This means that they are all in their raw form without chemicals, additives and processing. In basic terms you get more out your food when it is consumed in this way. This is because raw food contains more vital nutrients such as vitamins, antioxidants and amino acids. These are so good for your body that people who start eating them can experience a natural high as they are rapidly used up and turned into valuable materials. This means that green smoothies make you feel good as well as doing good.

Green smoothies are a valuable tool when it comes to dieting and losing weight. Due to the fact that they can make you feel fuller for longer they can help you to rapidly lose weight. They can also be the answer to the dieting plateau that many people reach on a normal low calorie diet. There are many other ways that green smoothies can enhance a diet or help in losing weight.

Green Smoothies could be your body's answer to those niggling health problems that can make life a misery. Modern life itself can have a bad effect on the human body and that includes the food that we eat. In seems that the further that we get away from nature, the more problems that we appear to have. If you look back to our ancestors they didn't have supermarkets and chemical additives to preserve and enhance the flavours and appearance of the foods they ate. You have to ask yourself how much damage all of these chemical additives cause? In addition to this even cooking foods causes chemical changes to happen to food and this can result in substances forming which can be bad for us and can even cause certain cancers.

If you feel like life is getting on top of you after too many 'little indulgencies' then green smoothies can be used as a way of detoxifying the body and rapidly returning it to normality.

Green Smoothie provides you with all of the information that you need to get your body working as nature intended. Get the book and join in this exciting new world of health.

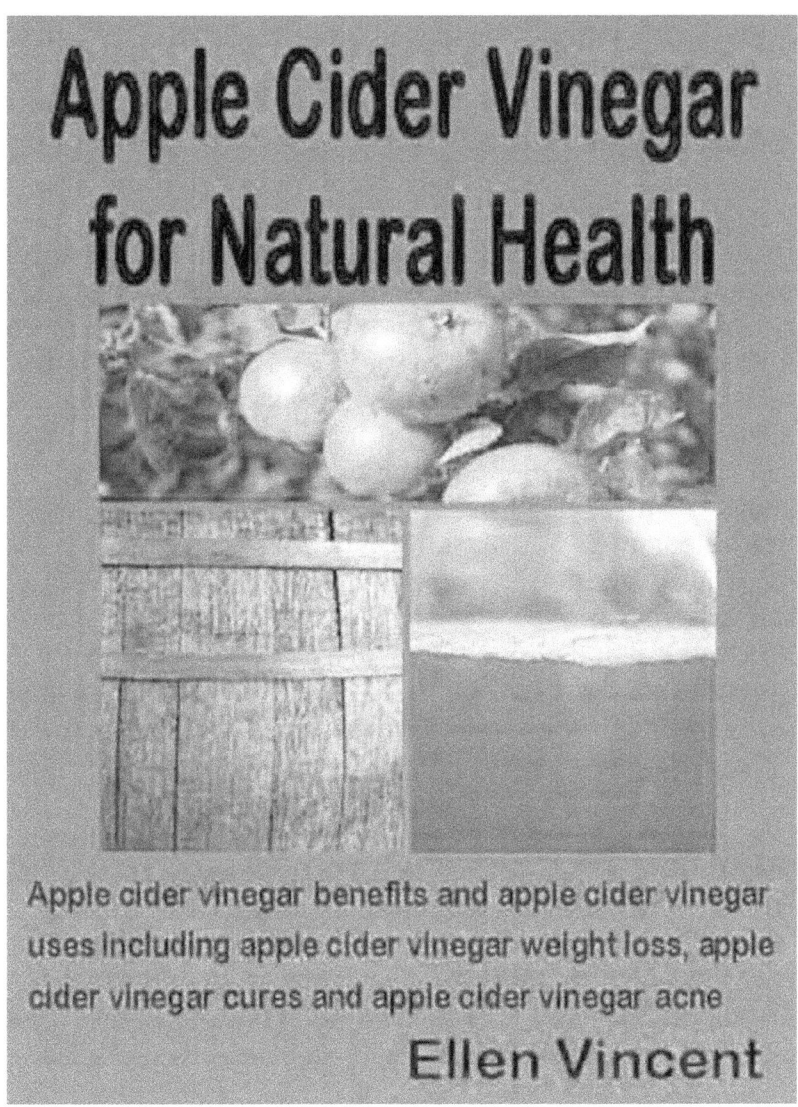

Kindle edition: http://www.amazon.com/Apple-Vinegar-Natural-Health-ebook/dp/B0076AAV6U/

Paperback: http://www.amazon.com/Apple-Cider-Vinegar-Natural-Health/dp/1475220707/

Apple cider vinegar for natural health is all about how you can use this wonderful natural health tonic to improve your life. Apple cider vinegar has been used for centuries to treat a whole host of illnesses and conditions. These cures and remedies have become part of our folklore, but that doesn't mean that we shouldn't take them seriously. Apple cider vinegar contains many health giving substances such as vitamins, minerals, antioxidants, bioflavenoids and of course the main ingredient of acetic acid. All of these things can help our bodies to work to the peak of performance and shrug off some of those day to day conditions that get us down. You can drink apple cider vinegar or apply it directly to the skin or hair. Either way you are getting the benefit of all of these super nutrients. Some books on apple cider vinegar are written by the people who are then trying to sell the vinegar to you. I am not involved in selling these products at all. My main interest comes from my scientific and educational background together with the fact that I use apple cider vinegar myself on many occasions during my day to day life. I am a real fan and take a daily tonic to ward off illness. I also use it on my skin and hair to great effect. I am so impressed with the results that I get with apple cider vinegar that I felt compelled to research it further and then write this book. I have never come across one single substance with so many uses before, and the results can often be stunning. So, take while and look at the information in the book and then try apple cider vinegar for yourself. Pretty soon you could become a real fan too!

This version 2 of the book contains extra information, and in particular details about how to use apple cider vinegar in your daily cooking. There are plenty of recipes and cookery ideas that you can try out for yourself.

Green Smoothie Recipes

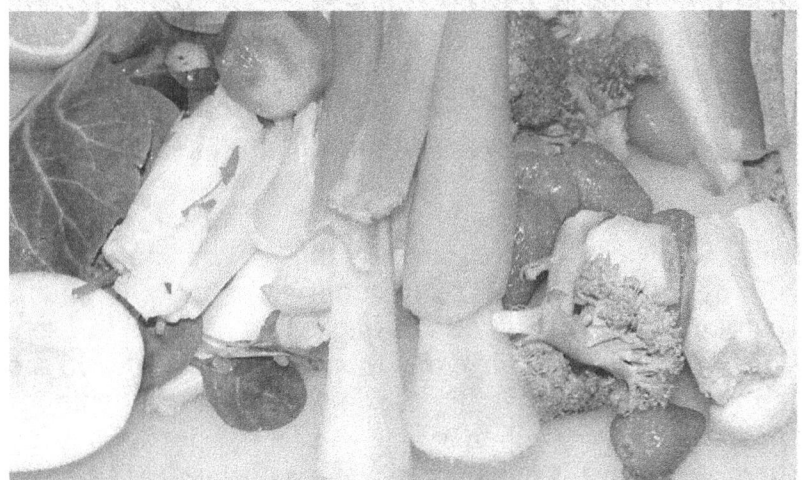

Over 200 green smoothie recipes fully indexed, with ingredients and amounts and grouped under the main green ingredient used

Ellen Vincent

Kindle edition: http://www.amazon.com/Green-smoothie-recipes-ingredients-ebook/dp/B009R4RQQG/

Paperback: http://www.amazon.com/Green-Smoothie-Recipes-ingredients-ingredient/dp/1480124117/

Green Smoothie Recipes gives you exactly what you want. Over 200 fully indexed green smoothies recipes with the amounts of everything that you need. Each recipe for green smoothie is grouped in chapters under the main green ingredient that is used. Every green smoothie recipe can be accessed individually by clicking a link on the contents page. Each of the chapter groups starts with the simplest recipes using the least ingredients and progresses up to more complicated ones at the end of each chapter. This way you can select a recipe that suits your needs and experience in making healthy green smoothies.

This book doesn't contain any fluff about the health benefits of drinking a green smoothie or the equipment that you need. It is assumed that you know how to use a blender and already have one that will successfully do the job. It also assumes that you are quite capable of throwing the ingredients into a blender and whizzing them up. There are no personal accounts detailing life changing events caused by drinking green smoothies. If you just need a whole lot of different healthy green smoothie recipes to keep you going and make your life more interesting then this is the book for you!

The best green smoothie will only have fruit and greens in it and won't have additives such as protein powders. Fresh ingredients are used in all of these raw green smoothie recipes. Included are green smoothie weight loss recipes, green smoothie diet recipes and detox smoothie recipes. Once you get started with all of these green smoothie recipes you will just want to carry on, experiment and create your own.

www.ingramcontent.com/pod-product-compliance
Lightning Source LLC
Chambersburg PA
CBHW070552290526
45790CB00002B/649